About the Author

David Grant studied at the Royal Veterinary College, London University, and Edinburgh University. He worked on a farm practice when he first qualified, and then at the RSPCA Harmsworth hospital as a junior vet. After a year in Colombia he only just survived the culture shock of working as a vet in Chelsea. He has been director of the RSPCA Harmsworth hospital since 1987. He is married with two children and lives in London.

Still Practising
From Country Vet to the Animal Hospital

DAVID GRANT

POCKET
BOOKS

LONDON · SYDNEY · NEW YORK · TOKYO · SINGAPORE · TORONTO

First published in Great Britain by Simon & Schuster UK Ltd, 2000
This edition first published by Pocket Books, 2001
An imprint of Simon & Schuster UK Ltd
A Viacom company

1 3 5 7 9 10 8 6 4 2

Simon & Schuster UK Ltd
Africa House
64–78 Kingsway
London WC2B 6AH

Simon & Schuster Australia
Sydney

A CIP catalogue record for this book is available
from the British Library

ISBN 0-7434-0902-7

Typeset by SX Composing DTP, Rayleigh, Essex
Printed and bound in Great Britain by
Omnia Books Ltd, Glasgow

Although all the stories that feature in this book are true, the names of
pets and owners have been changed to protect their privacy.

To Rachel

Acknowledgements

With thanks to Helen Gummer, Katharine Young, Robert Rimmer, Glen Saville and all the staff at Simon & Schuster. Special thanks go to Pepsy Dening and Julian Alexander.

Chapter One

Like so many other farms I had come to know since joining the practice eighteen months before, these ancient buildings buried deep in the Kentish countryside looked as if they hadn't been touched in five hundred years. The white-painted weather boarding, the russet of the brick walls and tiled roofs – it was as if time stood still, I thought, as I crossed the yard to the barn where my patient would be waiting. Once over the threshold, I became aware of the muffled sound of cows breathing. Then I saw her. Not my patient, but a girl sitting on a low stool, hair pushed into a cap, her arms moving in perfect rhythm as she pulled on the teats of a fine Friesian. Now this was strange. Some of the farms in the practice were pretty basic, but to my knowledge they all had milking parlours – perhaps the machine had broken down. As my eyes grew accustomed to the light I saw she was wearing a skirt that was pushed up over her knees and beneath it were wooden clogs.

I couldn't believe my luck – a real milkmaid! As I moved towards her, the noise of the milk ringing down rhythmically into the pail grew louder and louder, louder and louder.

Then with a start I woke up and reached for the phone. 'David?'

For a moment I didn't recognize the voice. I wasn't on call, that much I did know. When you're on call you sleep in a different way, only half asleep, alert for the slightest noise. But after the skinful I'd had the night before, I was as alert as a slug.

'It's Nick. Sorry to wake you but you said I could call in an emergency. The thing is a farmer called Roy Gibbons has a cow with a teat that needs stitching. And I just don't think I can handle it on my own.'

I groaned, told him he'd just ruined my chances of a meaningful relationship with a milkmaid, and said I'd meet him at the Gibbonses' place in thirty minutes. I groped for the light switch and wished I hadn't switched off the part of my brain which would have told me I'd had enough to drink before I agreed to that last pint.

Nick Lightfoot was the new boy at the practice, and yes, I had told him he could call me. He had been brought in on the small-animal side three weeks ago. This was his first night duty and, yes he was right, stitching a torn teat on a cow that big is not a one-man job.

When I arrived in Canterbury as assistant to the farm-animal team eighteen months before, I had little idea that the practice was due to expand. I don't even think the partners knew. But it was the tail end of the sixties, an era that had brought increased prosperity to everyone and as always happens in those circumstances, people were inclined to spend more on their pets, so that side of the practice was expanding. The previous summer the two partners specializing in domestic animals had been working under constant pressure while the three of us on the farm-animal side were having it relatively easy – except at night. It was a shift that foreshadowed the crises that were to beset agriculture in the second half of the century. Thirty years later the practice would lose its large-animal component altogether as one by one farmers got out of food animals, with the exception of a few giant concerns.

Still Practising

So the partners had decided the practice could afford another assistant to add to the small-animal team. I must admit that Nick Lightfoot had seemed a strange choice: he had no experience of small animals but was a high-flying academic who had just got his PhD in cardiology.

Although we were like chalk and cheese I had taken to him from the start. Like me Nick was a townie, but there the similarity ended. In common with the majority of vets in those days he was a product of the public-school system, with all the confidence that seemed to come with it, while I was a grammar-school boy with no confidence whatsoever. His father was a surgeon, mine a factory foreman. However, in spite of Nick's parentage and his blue-chip academic credentials I never felt threatened or in awe of him. Eighteen months on the job had made me realize that experience and common sense are worth any amount of qualifications.

As Nick reminded me when I asked why he'd gone for such a rural practice, the senior partners, Frank Archer and Alan Jenkins, were two of the most respected names in the veterinary world and an apprenticeship with them would give him the best possible practical background for a career as an academic, which was what he was aiming for. And Canterbury was near enough to London, and the practice big and go-ahead by the standards of the day – a hospital, with a fully equipped laboratory, operating theatre and X-ray room. From the start Nick knew where he was going: he would eventually become a world authority on the heart.

Roy Gibbons' farm lay deep in the Kentish Weald to the south-west of the city. The sky was just beginning to streak orange and red with the promise of daybreak when I checked the boot of my six-month old Ford Anglia – the veterinary equivalent of a doctor's bag – and started up the engine. Although the road ahead was still pitch dark – no leaking light from cities back then – I could see the sky turn gold in my rear-view mirror as I neared the farm.

'Well, blow me, David. You too? Don't tell Alan or he'll be charging me double!' However rough I felt, the sight of Roy's jovial face immediately cheered me up. Around fifty, I suppose, the area around his eyes was deeply etched, not from worry but from smiling. With one hand on mine and the other on my elbow Roy gave my hand a vigorous shaking which did nothing for the queasiness that seemed to have supplanted the headache the day had started with.

I smiled wanly. Roy turned his attention to Nick, who had arrived a few minutes before me and who was just pulling on his waders.

'As David will tell you once he regains the power of speech, I don't drink myself, and if ever I were tempted, the memory of young David here this morning would stop me in my tracks.' His laugh rang out across the farmyard and was answered by the morning's first cock crow.

Over the preceding year Roy had become a real friend. His lead cow Agnes had crossed my path on a number of occasions with – in retrospect – hilarious consequences. He had been a bomber pilot in the war and, although from the north originally, had decided to settle close to where he had been stationed.

Roy had a medium-sized herd of about fifty Friesians, but they were some of the biggest cows I had ever seen and by no means the tamest.

This time the patient wasn't Agnes but another hefty specimen called Patience. As we entered the cowshed she was munching the remains of her food concentrate, known locally as cake, and, true to her name, didn't seem too concerned about the gash in her teat. However I knew it would be a different story if anyone tried to touch it.

I've seen cows kick out at a fly if it dared to land on them and we would need to stay well clear until she was safely tethered if a good kicking was to be avoided. A close inspection of the wound would have to wait until the area was safely anaesthetized. But first there was the problem of injecting the anaesthetic.

These days there are sedative injections but the only way then to prevent a cow kicking was to hold up one of the front legs or to push the tail up so that it was nearly vertical – preferably both. So Roy looped a rope around her front leg and hoisted it up over a partition so that it worked as a pulley, an old farmer's trick that means you hardly need use any effort, while I took up position at the rear.

Nick and I had agreed that my role on this occasion was as muscle and moral support, and that he should do everything else. First came the anaesthetic, a ring block around the base of the teat, five separate injections with a very fine needle, while I held the tail up and Roy held the rope. The five-minute wait while the anaesthetic took effect was enlivened by Roy regaling Nick with the history of Agnes and her uncanny ability to cover either me or my car with dung.

The next step was to clean up the wound and see the extent of the damage. It turned out to be a bad gash. But before stitching a teat siphon had to be inserted so that the milk could continue to be drawn off. Roy would have to keep it sterilized for use every time she was milked.

Stitching up an animal that is awake is very different from stitching up one that is asleep and lying on a table. The anaesthetic might have numbed her teat, but it didn't stop her shifting around from foot to foot.

'This is worse than trying to lace a shoe while the owner is tap dancing,' said Nick between cutting one stitch and beginning the next.

'I see you've got a sense of humour on you, young man,' said Roy. 'It will stand you in good stead round here, mark my words.'

And he was right. My own acceptance into the farming community had less to do with my ability to cure animals than an ability to hold my drink and take a joke, something which I had demonstrated at the farmers' Christmas shindig the year I arrived, when the prime motive was to separate the goats from the sheep by springing a surprise on the new vet. To the delight of all concerned, I turned out to be a goat.

Stitching up a teat is always a long job but considering this was the first time that Nick had ever attempted anything like it on a real-life cow, he managed the stitch-up quite deftly. Not bad for an academic, I thought. It took half an hour and ten stitches.

By the time we had finished with Patience the sun was up and the milking parlour was in full hum under the capable eye of George, Roy's head herdsman.

'Dare say you've got time for breakfast, boys.'

Nick's face lit up. A farm breakfast is a perk that small-animal vets rarely experience.

'Gosh, jolly kind of you, sir.'

'Now don't you go sirring me. Getting you out in the middle of the night it's the least I can do. Though I'm not sure your pal here is up to it,' he added slapping my back with a hearty laugh.

While Nick got cleaned up, I chatted to Roy about Julie, the Gibbonses' lovely daughter, who had just finished her first year as a student nurse. Then it was my turn in the bathroom. The sight that met me in the mirror explained a lot. I looked absolutely dreadful, and about ten years older than Nick, though in fact he was a year older than me.

When I got back to the kitchen, Roy's wife, Katherine, was standing with her back to the Aga, still in her dressing gown. It was the first time I had seen her with her brown and grey hair down, hair that she wore up during the day. Roy and Nick were nowhere to be seen.

'Your young friend saw a couple of mushrooms on the dresser that Roy picked yesterday,' Katherine explained. 'Roy said he thought there would be more after last night's rain. So they've gone out mushrooming like a couple of big kids. Goodness knows when they'll be back. So I've put everything in the lower oven to keep warm. I'm just going to get dressed, so I'm leaving you in charge, David, if that's all right. The tea's just brewed. So help yourself.'

It must have been about ten minutes before the 'big kids' came back, each with a white pudding basin overflowing with mushrooms, their gills still pink, barely hours old. These days cultivated mushrooms are everywhere, but in the sixties they were still a luxury and field mushrooms – as they still are – a real treat.

'I must tell you, David, you've got competition,' said Roy, as he wiped each mushroom with what looked like a freshly ironed linen handkerchief and gently eased it into a frying pan, black from years of use, sizzling with butter. 'Young Nick here was across those fields like a hare. And nothing of him either. What did you say your name was?' he said turning to Nick. 'Lightfoot? Well named. Extremely well named.'

So then the talk turned to running. Neither Nick nor I had realized the other was an athlete. Before this morning we had only met at the practice where the talk was of animals, but it turned out that Nick was a keen cross-country runner, whereas I, with a quite different, heavier build, was a sprinter. As we both tucked into poached eggs, bacon, fried bread and field-fresh mushrooms, Roy told Nick how the summer he had first met me I was always using his fields for training and how I'd have made the Olympic team if only I'd stuck at it.

'Don't take any notice of him,' I protested. 'These farmers – catch a cow and they think you're David Hemery.'

'So why didn't you?' Nick asked. 'Continue I mean.'

'It was either the running or the job,' I explained. 'Perhaps if I'd been on the small animal side like you, it might have been possible, but what with night duty and weekend duty, and sheer exhaustion, it was impossible to do both. And, in spite of what Roy might say the Olympics was never an option. But I was good county standard, the Kent 100 and 200 metres champion in my time. And I still go to the odd meeting. Nothing serious though.'

'Don't you miss competing?' Roy asked as he refilled our tea cups.

'The competing, well yes, sometimes I do. But not the training. And it's the training that takes all the time. I'm perfectly happy to chase cows and sheep. I'll leave chasing medals to others.'

As we left, Roy presented Nick with a sturdy paper carrier bag full of the remaining mushrooms – there were no plastic bags in those days. Nick had apparently told Roy that his wife was a great cook and would be jealous when he told her what he'd had for breakfast.

'Doing anything tonight?' Nick said, poking his head out of the Anglia window. As a small-animal assistant, he didn't get a car of his own and this was the practice spare, my old grey mare.

'I'm on call,' I sighed.

'But you don't have to be at your place, do you?'

'No, but . . .'

'And you still have to eat. So come round to us and I'll put Selina through her paces. God knows I owe you. Don't forget I ruined your chances of a meaningful relationship with a milkmaid.'

I laughed. 'But hadn't you better ask your wife first?'

'This isn't a dinner party you idiot, this is kitchen supper, and as you're providing half the ingredients she's hardly going to object. So. See you at, what, half seven?'

And with that he revved off the dial and spun out of the gate, throwing up an arc of mud that completely spattered my windscreen. Behind me Roy roared with laughter as I threw a bucket of water at it and had to get more to clean my waders.

'Green as they come. You were as bad, David. But we'll make a vet of him yet.'

I had no more sleep that night and the prospect of another long night in front of me. Thankfully all I had booked in for the day was a routine test for tuberculosis, known as a TT test, at a large farm down on the marshes, all that's left of the sea that once separated the Isle of Thanet from the mainland of Kent. It lasted all day but didn't take too much out of me – no decisions to be taken, no life and death situations to contend with. And considering my lack of sleep, I found myself looking forward to meeting Nick's wife.

As I was on call I drove to the address he'd given me, although it was less than ten minutes' walk away from the hospital, and parked in the narrow street in the shadow of the great wall that rings Canterbury like a stone moat.

From the moment she opened the door to me that evening I knew that Selina Lightfoot was cast from a different mould than any other girls I had known. She was funny and forthright and said exactly what she thought.

'Welcome to the madhouse,' she said, 'you must be David.' And she gave me a peck on the cheek, not common practice in those days, even if you knew someone well. It quite took me aback; I had never even seen her before.

'Did Nick ask you to bring a bottle?'

'No, but . . .' and I handed her one I had picked up at the local off-licence.

'You're a sweetheart David. Nick said I would like you and he was right. Now follow me. Oh, my name's Selina by the way.'

We went through the sitting room into the kitchen. It was a small terraced house that had been extended at the back. From the ceiling hung pots and pans, sieves, jugs, ladles, mallets, tongs, all suspended from butchers' hooks. They had only been there three weeks, but it felt more like a home than my flat at the Nightingales', where I had lived for eighteen months. Nick was nowhere to be seen.

Selina reached up to a hook and passed me a corkscrew.

'You do it, you're stronger than me.' I dutifully uncorked the bottle I was holding.

'Now,' she said, grabbing two glasses, 'We'll try yours first and then mine.'

An inch of red wine went into each glass. She swirled it round, sniffed it, then drank it. Or rather gargled while I stood mesmerized. She had the most wonderful hair, which always moved more slowly than she did, consequently it was constantly falling half across her face and she'd have to push it back, so shiny it could have been used in a Silvikrin advert.

Still Practising

'Come on, hurry up,' she spluttered as she tried to keep the wine in her mouth. 'Now the next one.' She passed another already opened bottle of wine from beside the stove. Another inch. Another swill and swig.

'So what do you think?'

'How do you mean?'

'Which one is better? Which would you rather drink? I need one bottle to go in the *coq au vin* and didn't want to put mine in if yours was worse. If Nick were here it wouldn't be so bad. He knows about wine. I mean he understands labels. But I don't. They're all the same to me.'

'Where is he?'

'Being a good neighbour I think. But stop changing the subject. At this rate we won't eat until midnight. Which one?'

'Well the man in the shop said this was a good vintage.'

It had cost me 19s 11d in old money, just a penny under £1, a twentieth of my weekly take home pay, but I didn't know much about wine; beer was more my territory.

'So you think yours is better then?'

'Well, not exactly,' I said, adding diplomatically 'in fact I think yours is rather nicer.'

'Good,' she said. 'I like a man who can make a decision. So that's that. We'll drink ours and cook with yours.'

And with that she emptied the contents of the bottle I had brought into a casserole and put it into the oven.

'Now we can relax. Gin and tonic?'

I explained that I was on call so I would limit myself to one glass of wine with the meal.

Just then Nick burst in. 'Sorry, David. Some poor bugger with a flat battery. Hope Selina explained. I was just coming back from my run when I came across him so I gave him a jump start. My goodness,' he added, as he

11

stood at the sink washing his hands, 'this is damn good of you, David.'

'What is?'

'This bottle. 1962 Chateau Estephe. Cru Bourgeouis. Amazing. Didn't know you were a wine buff. We'll have him round again, won't we darling?'

I looked at Selina and she looked at me and our eyes both turned towards the oven.

Nick dried his hands on a tea towel.

'What did I say? Oh God, David. Of course. Bloody insensitive. You're on call. You won't be able to drink any of this nectar.'

'Neither will you honey bunch,' Selina chipped in, knowing the truth had to come out. 'Although you may get to eat it,' she giggled, up-ending the empty bottle onto the draining board where a few sad dregs dripped out. 'I predict that this will be the best *coq au vin* you have ever tasted.'

There followed a split second of embarrassed silence, then simultaneously we all roared with laughter, the ice, if there ever was any, well and truly broken.

As they busied themselves with laying the table with an extraordinary mixture of junk-shop plates, each one a different pattern, I watched their easy familiarity enviously, thinking sadly of what might have been, with Sally and even with Angie. They clearly adored each other, though to look at they made a slightly unconventional couple. Nick was a good bit shorter than me while Selina was taller than the average girl. He was as thin as a whippet while she was sultry: voluptuous and olive-skinned, like a young Sophia Loren. The only feature they shared was curly hair, although hers was black and his was choir-boy golden. But from the start it was clear that they were true soul mates.

'How much did you pay for tonight's gravy, David?'

Still Practising

Nineteen and eleven was more than I usually paid, but not by much. Nick whistled.

'A bargain. So that's all right then. It's half the price it should have been.' Behind him Selina was doing a don't-take-any-notice-of-him mime. 'These little off-licences sometimes have bottles like this hanging around for years and they never put the price up. So I'll get round there in the morning and buy up what they've got and just hope it wasn't the last bottle. Imagine, if this hadn't happened we'd never have found out. Anyway, it only means that you'll have to come back to see just what we missed this evening.'

I said that it hadn't tasted that special, but that didn't impress him. A wine of that quality, he assured me, had to breathe for at least an hour before you had any chance of judging it properly. What I knew about wine could be written on a cork, however. White with fish, red with meat.

The smells coming from the kitchen were now irresistible. The house was rented – they had been married for less than a year – and they already knew that Kent was just a stepping stone on Nick's career path. Selina was a primary-school teacher and had no difficulty getting a job in Canterbury. And that kind of teaching, she pointed out, she could do anywhere. They planned to stay two years.

I knew by now that I was in for something special in the culinary line. I rarely had anything more adventurous than beans on toast or bacon and egg back at my flat. To build up the necessary daily calorie intake I usually went to a restaurant opposite the Cathedral called Peggoty's Pantry, where they did a three-course 'business' lunch – soup, meat and four veg and sweet for 3s. A cup of tea or instant coffee was 6d extra. Dickens wrote *David Copperfield* when he was living in Canterbury, a fact that had not been forgotten by the tourist trade, hence the name Peggoty's Pantry. The

13

building, with its overhanging upper floors was old even when Dickens was alive; Chaucer, that other favourite when it came to naming cafés, could have supped there. However the regularity of my visits had nothing to do with its historical connections or the food, and everything to do with one of the waitresses.

The two waitresses both wore the same uniform of black skirt and starched white pinny. In size they were like Laurel and Hardy. The chief one was about forty I suppose – she had two children at secondary school and a husband who worked for the fire brigade. Her skirt reached to her knees but was always gaping around the zip. Needless to say it was the other waitress I was interested in. If Caroline's skirt had been any shorter it wouldn't have justified the name of skirt at all, which probably accounted for the army of lunchtime regulars, male like me but, unlike me, old enough to be her father.

Selina certainly lived up to her reputation. The first course, naturally, was stuffed mushrooms, really meaty and crusty on the top with garlic bread crumbs and parsley. I had never had anything like it. We had three each, the size of beer mats. Then after a suitable pause, during which we discussed my love life, came the *coq au vin*. I don't know what it would have tasted like with ordinary plonk, but this was amazing. She must have spent hours peeling dozens of whole onions smaller than gobstoppers (my favourite sweet when I was a boy) and of course this was where the smaller mushrooms ended up. It was served with what she called *pommes dauphinoise*, wafer-thin slices of potato baked with cream and served with a green salad. All very French. To finish we had something called floating islands – meringues floating in what Selina told me was custard, not that it resembled anything I'd ever had called custard. At home my mother always insisted on Birds (there were some cheaper powdered brands she didn't approve of). Selina's custard had never seen a tin but was made from egg yolks and boiling milk and sugar. It was out of this world. The meal was finished off with Camembert – the first time I had had it. She had found it she told me in a small grocer's called Milsoms that stocked French cheeses in one of Canterbury's many narrow side streets. Did I know it? I didn't like to admit that the only things my store cupboard ran to were cans of Double Diamond and baked beans. At first I was a bit tentative, but encouraged by Selina's gentle ribbing along the lines of how I must be used to farmyard smells, this was the chance to actually taste them, I was immediately a convert.

When the subject of my own love life had come up I had given them a brief run-down on my four-year relationship with Sally, whom I had met while I was at university, which had ended because I was here and she was in London, and on my nine-month non-relationship with Angie, one of the ten female students who lived at the house where I had my flat, which had ground to a halt because I couldn't give her what she wanted. Commitment.

'But what about now?' Selina pressed.

Reluctantly I admitted that David Grant was a romance-free zone.

'Well, that's got to change. Look at you! What girl could resist such a strapping Adonis? Nick and you are like the before and after pictures in an advertisement for body building. Can't think what I see in him,' she said, looking at her husband adoringly and ruffling his hair.

'Seriously Selina, the problem is that I just seem to muck things up. I'm just no good at this commitment thing. I get involved with really nice girls, really nice. But – I

15

don't know. I suppose I think that there will be some kind of lightening flash that will tell me this is the one. And that's never happened. So they just get fed up and leave.'

'That's because you haven't met the right girl,' she insisted, wagging a finger at me.

'Selina's right,' added Nick. 'And in order to meet the right one, you have to meet lots of them. It's what a marketing friend of mine calls the numbers game. We're always having Selina's girlfriends to stay.' Then turning back to his wife added, 'Talking of which, isn't Kiki coming some time soon?'

Selina's eyes seemed to double in size.

'Of course. You're a genius, husband of mine.'

'Well, David,' explained Nick, 'you're in luck. Selina's friend Kiki is a real cracker and comes complete with a full set of limbs and other female characteristics that, if I weren't married to the most gorgeous girl in the world, might even turn my head.' It turned out that she was an actress, and coming to do an Italian comedy at the Marlowe Theatre in a couple of months' time.

The food was as intoxicating as alcohol and soon we were talking about the partners, which I suspected had been the original reason for the invitation. I realized that I had never talked with anyone like this. Although when I arrived at the practice there were only two partners, Frank Archer and Alan Jenkins, the two other vets were both rather remote. In fact Charles Harte and Peter Cooper were now up there on the letterhead with Frank and Alan. The only non-partners now were Nick and myself.

Selina had only met Peter, who together with Frank – and now Nick – made up the small-animal team. I hadn't had much to do with him. So I gave her a thumbnail sketch of the others: Frank had the energy of a teenager combined

Still Practising

with the wisdom of Solomon. Gave the impression of being a bit of a boffin – with a bow tie to give the right touch of eccentricity. Frank had started as a farm animal vet but now worked exclusively in the hospital, except when called out for emergencies. Partner or not, everyone had to do night duty.

Alan was quite different. A former county rugby player, he always looked impeccable – dark suit, dark tie, handkerchief in his top pocket. Welsh in every way except his accent which was public school pukka. His nod to eccentricity was a flower in his buttonhole, which could be anything from a rose to a daffodil. I even remember a sprig of wild cherry blossom he picked from a hedgerow when we were out together.

Both Frank and Alan shared a keen intelligence and were expert in giving off-the-cuff seminars to apprentices who hadn't a clue what they were doing – and their fuses could at times be very short indeed.

I had directed all this at Selina, who was sitting beside me. Opposite me, Nick had been quietly listening. He had now had three weeks at the practice. Had my guided tour around the partners been about right? Nick nodded and laughed. 'Well, so far they've all been amazingly kind and helpful.'

'The important bit of that sentence is "so far",' I replied. 'You just wait till the honeymoon is over, your view might change then.'

'And what about that young upstart Grant. Think I'll have trouble with him? A farmer I met today warned me that he was a bad influence, a bit of a secret toper, and that I should steer well clear.'

'Oh I quite agree,' I said, warming to the game, 'he's a terror. Knows nothing about wine, terrible cook. Though he

17

could write a book about pubs and beer. But whatever you do, never ever call him out at night, unless you want to invite him to dinner the next day.'

It was midnight by the time I left. Although it was late September and there was a real sense of autumn in the air, it felt like spring, like a new beginning. Although I didn't know it at the time, in Selina and Nick Lightfoot I had found lifelong friends.

The last nine months living at Mrs Nightingale's had not been easy. Any idea I might have had that Angie and I could be friends had proved impossible. My feelings towards her had not changed, nor I think had hers for me. But she wanted more than I could give. Anything less she seemed to see as some kind of rejection. What made it really difficult was that we still lived only yards apart. I knew Mrs Nightingale thought I had behaved badly and after Angie and I had split up, the invitations to meals had definitely dried up. Yet living in the same building – although with quite separate entrances – meant I didn't feel I could get involved with anybody else. And who else was there anyway? The only girls I met were the girls in the house, all students at the same teacher-training college. So by the time they left for the holidays in July my love life had reached an all time low.

But Angie's departure from Canterbury at the end of the summer term had triggered some kind of release mechanism and it wasn't long afterwards that the old hormones had begun to make their presence felt.

When I had told Nick and Selina that David Grant was a romance-free zone, I had not been entirely honest. At the end of August I had finally plucked up enough courage to ask the waitress at Peggoty's Pantry out to the pictures. She was studying French at London University and it was just a holiday job. Caroline had long red hair, and her face was covered with freckles. She wasn't conventionally pretty but sometimes – even discounting the black mini skirt – she was truly beautiful, particularly if you saw her in profile, with the sun streaming in the plate-glass window of the restaurant.

Perhaps because Caroline and I had not had not met in a 'romantic' context, I never felt ill at ease with her and gradually we began to chat. Although the restaurant was opposite the Cathedral, it wasn't really a tourist place, but was used by people working in the town and her regulars, the 'old men' as I called them, had usually gone by two. Joan, the other waitress would disappear back into the kitchens, so we had the place to ourselves.

There was always a small poster advertising films at the local cinema hanging beside the cash register and one day I had plucked up courage and asked if she'd seen the latest James Bond film, which were as popular then as they are today. She said no. Would she like to see it? Yes. We went the following evening.

It was still early days, she hadn't yet been back to the flat, but that was about to be remedied and I had planned a little tête-à-tête for the coming weekend. For once the fridge was full, although after tonight's meal my planned offering of *chilli con carne* seemed a little lacking in appeal.

I knew I shouldn't get my hopes up too high; it could just turn out to be a re-run of the Sally story: in a couple of weeks she was due to go back to university in London, and I would be stuck here. Then I remembered Kiki. An actress. Hmmm. I went to sleep with a smile on my face, barely even aware that I was on call.

Chapter Two

I may have forgotten I was on call, but Frank hadn't. At 4.30 in the morning the phone rang, and this time I awoke at the first ring. Milk fever out on the coast, no time to waste. Milk fever, though easy to cure, is a life-and-death matter. Ted Knight had recently come onto the practice books. I'd only been out to him once before and he seemed reasonable enough: a red-faced man in his late forties with a quiet manner. He weighed up everything before he spoke, which at first made me think of him as innately suspicious of us 'vet'in'ries'. But he seemed satisfied with my efforts and Frank's wife, who had taken the call, said he even asked her 'if that young fella Grant would be coming' .

It was raining again and the windscreen wipers of the Anglia were barely able to keep pace. In order to wake myself up I tuned in to Radio Caroline, the original offshore pirate radio station. Although the BBC had recently brought in Radio 1 – along the lines of 'if you can't beat 'em, join 'em' – Radio Caroline was still the only place you could hear anything in the middle of the night. At least the roads were straight going this way and I could get up a bit of speed, not like the twists and turns of last night's route into the Weald.

I put the Anglia into top gear and hurtled down the straight country lane towards Ted Knight's farm about 10 miles distant. I turned the radio up as loud as it would go in order to drown out the noise of the windscreen wipers. It was Louis Armstrong's 'It's A Wonderful World', an old standard which he was making into a hit second time around. And it was a wonderful world, at least mine was, though I could have done without a milk fever at five in the morning. With this rain there was no way I would avoid a soaking; at least last night's gashed teat had been under cover.

Milk fever is a condition caused by very low calcium and happens soon after calving. The cow goes down and can't get up, and it will die without treatment. Luckily it's very simple to cure – a bottle of calcium borogluconate injected into the vein often results in a 'miraculous' cure. Ted Knight didn't know how long she had been down before he found her. It seemed he had been alerted by his dog.

The Anglia, with its raked-backed rear window, might look like something from *Thunderbirds*, I reflected, but as the speedometer touched 70 mph, no one could complain at the little car's engine. At this rate I would be there in about five minutes.

In my daydreaming I had been completely unaware of a car following me. A sudden cacophony of sound and a flashing blue light was a very rude awakening. I pulled over with a pounding heart, all atremble.

A young WPC motioned me to wind down the window. She looked even younger than me – a young twenty five – maybe even a year or so less. Her companion was just as young-looking, a stringy gangling teenager with a spotty face, wearing a cap that was two sizes two big for him. A third whose face I couldn't see was still at the wheel of the panda car – presumably all set to give chase in case I decided to make a break for it. They were not happy.

'In a hurry, sir?' The young WPC looked at me with

barely suppressed glee in anticipation of making me crawl as she filled out the inevitable ticket.

'Well, yes I am rather. I'm a vet. I've been called out to an emergency. Life and death. Just past the next village.'

My smile, I hoped, conveyed just the right mix of friendliness and anxiety. From small babies, humans are programmed to respond to a smile. Try it some time. It is very hard not to smile if someone is smiling at you. She was an exception.

'I see, sir. Name?'

'David Grant. Like I said . . .'

'Would you mind stepping out of the car, sir.'

'Look officer, I'm serious. If you don't believe me, look in the boot.'

'That may be, sir. But if you'd be so kind as to get out of the car I would like you to blow into this bag.'

The 'breathalyser' as it was called had recently been introduced by Barbara Castle, the Labour Minister of Transport.

'But I'm on call. I haven't had a drink in the last twenty-four hours.'

'I'll be the judge of that.'

I got out of the car, aware that the minutes were ticking away and the chances of my reaching the downed cow in time were getting smaller and smaller. There seemed nothing for it but to blow into the bag through a rather unpleasant-looking plastic straw. I wouldn't have minded so much if it had been administered by the WPC, but it was the spotty youth. Out of the corner of my eye I noticed that the WPC was looking at the vast array of equipment and drugs necessary to ply my trade with more than a cursory interest. I suddenly saw a chink of light in this sorry scenario. It was a wild card, but worth a chance.

'Look, I know this is a lot to ask but I'm nearly there, and it really is an emergency and frankly I could do with a hand.'

She took the bait – although I sensed she wasn't out of the water yet. Within less than a minute we were underway – going at well over the speed limit, I should add. Less than three minutes later the convoy arrived at a bemused Ted Knight's farm.

'I didn't ask for the law as well – I hope there's no extra charge!' The farmer looked quite taken aback, I didn't know if he meant it or it was a joke.

'All part of the service – I needed to get here quickly. The officers were kind enough to escort me. Where's the cow?'

'She's gone down in the field near to the parlour – didn't quite make it home.'

A few minutes later, armed with the bottle of calcium, drip set and needles and a powerful police torch, we arrived at the patient.

As soon as she saw Betsy, the tough WPC became a tearful softy as she looked at the collapsed cow groaning, her breath coming in rasps and occasionally making desperate attempts to get up. The young woman dropped to her knees and tried to comfort her. The quickest way in was via the jugular. Quickly I hooked a rope around Betsy's neck and found the vein, and within a few minutes the calcium solution was flowing in with the gangling youth holding the bottle and his colleague talking all the time to the patient, smiling up at me as Betsy's distress diminished.

Meanwhile I sat on Betsy's back and waited for the inevitable improvement. With a few hundred of these cases under my belt now, I had amassed not only a lot of experience but a lot of confidence too. I had time to look at

David Grant

the young WPC, who by now I knew was called Rose. In this light she suddenly looked vulnerable and pretty. She glanced up, catching me admiring her and then turned away to hide a blush that she couldn't hide even in torch light.

'Will she be all right?'

'Absolutely. In fact in a minute you may have to get out of the way in case she tries to get up. And as for you,' I said turning to the gangly youth, 'you'd better watch out. One of the signs of recovery from milk fever is passing a large motion.' For a fleeting moment I had the pleasure of watching this cocky young man look distinctly worried.

It took ten minutes for the bottle to empty. Would I still get a ticket? I had one last trump card to play, though I'd have to be careful with the phrasing.

'I think I've met a colleague of yours. I'm a good friend of his daughter's.'

'What's his name?'

'Ken Hitchens.'

Both of them laughed out loud.

'Good job it wasn't Ken who stopped you,' chortled the youth. Sixty mph in a 40 mph area, he'd have you nicked, emergency or no emergency. He never lets anyone off.'

'Does that mean I'm off the hook then – err – officers,' I added with belated deference.

Before they could reply our patient started to get up and I caught hold of the young policewoman and pulled her away. For a moment I had her in my arms and we both laughed.

She looked at her sidekick. 'Verbal warning?'

He raised his eyes, then nodded with a resigned grin.

I breathed a sigh of relief. I already had a couple of points on my licence for speeding and they add up, and a vet without a licence is a vet without a job.

24

Then, as we were packing up Rose took me completely by surprise.

'I was wondering. I mean, I wouldn't want to be a bother, but, is there any chance I could come out with you?' She blushed, realizing what she had just said, and quickly added, 'I mean, on your rounds, or whatever you call it. On your calls . . . to farms . . . emergencies.' I stopped her before she got herself digging a deeper and deeper hole, I said that I wasn't sure if it was allowed.

Of course there was no rule about taking other people on a call – in fact the few times I had taken Angie out with me had always succeeded in bringing us closer. Perhaps that's what I was afraid of. Because, although it was early days, there was Caroline to consider. I didn't imagine she would take too kindly to an attractive young policewoman asking if she could come out on the rounds with me in her spare time. I said I'd ask the bosses, although I wasn't sure whether they would wear it. Nor, I imagined, would Caroline.

To say I knew her father was a bit of an exaggeration. It had been raining after our most recent trip to the cinema, so I had naturally offered to take Caroline home in the car. She lived in a modern estate on the edge of town with her parents and her younger sister. Why didn't I come in for a cup of coffee, she had suggested. Just as she took out her key the door had opened and a man with carrot red hair and in a policeman's uniform came out looking like thunder, gave me a glare and went straight to his car.

'What was all that about?' I had asked.

'Oh nothing. That's just Dad in a strop. He doesn't approve of me having boyfriends.'

Caroline's father!

'Don't worry,' she said, giving my nose a playful tweak.

Then added, 'He'll just take it out on some poor motorist like he always does. He's always in a better mood when he's been out on speed traps. One thing you can say about my dad. He loves his work.'

As I waved goodbye to the boys and girl in blue, the words and melody of the Louis Armstrong hit suddenly came flooding into my mind again. I didn't know so much about 'wonderful world'. 'Funny old world' suddenly seemed more appropriate. First Caroline, and now a WPC asking to come out with me. Having lived like a monk for the last year or so, opportunities to change the situation were suddenly popping up without my looking for them.

True to form, Ted Knight had said very little throughout the whole episode except for a grunt of satisfaction when he saw his cow get up. There would be no farm breakfast this time.

I slowly made my way back down the farm track to the road where I had been apprehended earlier and once back on the highway kept the speedometer at a steady forty. It didn't do to push your luck. The sun was up, and a beautiful day was in prospect. Last night's rain had left everything clean and fresh, although it had brought down the first of the autumn leaves. The rear-view mirror was filled with a huge red globe that seemed to be bouncing on the horizon like a balloon, and the whole sky was suffused with pink. I felt great, as I always did having done a good job and knowing there was probably time to have a full English breakfast before the morning rounds. I pulled into a transport café, the only car in a lorry park of juggernauts on their way to the ferry at Dover or Folkestone and settled down to a plate of eggs, bacon, sausage, Spam, chips and a fried slice all washed down with a mug of hot, sweet tea. On the blackboard behind the counter it was called the Last Breakfast, and written beside it was, 'Keeps you going till you get back.'

The morning's list wasn't too bad. First call was Chris Oliver, less than a mile from Roy Gibbons' place just over the North Downs. Chris and his wife Diana were newcomers to farming. Although Chris had been brought up on the farm it was only when his father died that, faced with the option of selling the place, he had decided to make a go of it himself. Diana had been a high-powered secretary but was now a farmer's wife.

My visit was a routine pregnancy diagnosis in one of the Olivers' small dairy herd. Most of my clients were small farmers. It was due to an ancient custom, unique to Kent, called Gavelkind. When William the Conqueror invaded in 1066, he allowed Kent to keep this old Saxon law, which said if there wasn't a will, property had to be divided between all the sons, not just given to the eldest, as became the custom everywhere else. It was only stopped in 1925. Over the centuries this has led to a patchwork of small farms. Because the land is so fertile, somehow they have survived.

Chris had a small herd of Ayrshires and I had two to inspect. From the hospital I took a short cut out of town, then headed south along the Roman road that sliced straight down across the county, singing along with The Foundations' jaunty hit single 'Build Me Up Buttercup' blaring out of the car radio. Its syncopated rhythm seemed to match the up-and-down nature of the road. A sharp right just before a small stand of oak trees that were just beginning to turn, and suddenly everything changed and there wasn't a straight stretch of tarmac to be seen. The Romans had laid their roads when the Weald was still forested. The people who cleared the land and eventually farmed it hadn't the Romans' single-mindedness. They went round any obstacles in their path, not up and over them. And so did I. Four miles of twists and turns, following the bend of a stream or the curve of a hill, and I was there.

As I walked over to the red tiled barn, I had a sudden sense of *déjà vu*. Then I remembered. The dream! But instead of a milkmaid sitting on a three-legged stool in a pool of sunlight, there was Chris filling in some Milk Marketing Board paperwork, with an old black Labrador, his muzzle nearly completely grey, lying beside him.

'So, which ones are they then?'

He motioned to two cows quietly munching on cake at the back of the barn. He looked tense. Did he know something I didn't? Then it was on with the protective clothing. At this early stage, the only way to tell if the cow was pregnant was to feel if the ovaries were enlarged, which meant putting my arm up her rectum and palpating the womb on the other side of the rectal wall. To find the ovaries you work your way up the uterus, find the 'horns' at the top, then you should feel them – two things about the size of golf balls – and also feel if the uterus seems enlarged. You are literally working in the dark. It is quite a skill, and was something I was still developing and was always a bit worried about, perhaps because I knew how important the outcome was, particularly to a small dairy farmer like Chris.

The whole purpose of getting a cow pregnant is to get milk from her. Keeping a cow's milk-yield high is a dairy farmer's number one priority. In normal circumstances a cow will provide milk over at least eight months. About thirty days after giving birth she comes into season – a good pointer is when you see cows trying to ride each other: the one doing the riding is nearly ready, and the one being ridden is a prime candidate for the artificial inseminator who will provide the best possible semen to ensure that the next generation is as high-yielding as possible. Near the end of the nine-month pregnancy the milk yield begins to drop off and the cow is 'dried off'. The cow gives birth every year and is almost constantly in milk. After seven or eight years of this, the cows themselves are clapped out. It's not an aspect of farming that I like.

Unlike sheep, cows calve throughout the year. Also unlike sheep, which usually give birth on their own, a cow's pregnancy is monitored nearly as closely as a human's, and the birth is rarely accomplished without someone around – the farmer if it's straightforward, the vet if there are complications.

The pregnancy is checked out between eight and twelve weeks. Because of the shape of the cow nothing shows before the last couple of months and it's important for the farmer to know well before that so he can start feeding her up or – if the artificial insemination hasn't worked – call in the ministry vet for a repeat visit.

Chris had positioned himself at the cow's head and I could see his face turned anxiously towards mine. His relief when I nodded and gave a thumbs up sign with my free hand was visible.

As I'd made good time coming down and there was no rush for my next call – just checking on some pigs I had recently vaccinated – I joined Chris and Di in the kitchen for a cup of coffee, not instant but percolated which had just started to be fashionable. Fashion and farmers don't usually go together but Di seemed determined to keep up with at least some of her city ways.

In spite of the good news about Dusty and Cilla – the Olivers showed more imagination that usual in naming their

cows, and sixties pop icons were as good as anything –
when I joined Chris in the kitchen after cleaning up, he was
looking tense again.

The reason, it turned out, was Monty, lying in his basket
and panting heavily. Monty was thirteen, old for a
Labrador, but he had belonged to Chris's father, who had
served with General Montgomery in the North Africa
campaign in the Second World War – hence the name – and
so there were a lot of emotions in play. As Chris tugged at
Monty's ears and massaged his head, I had a look at the old
dog. His abdomen was horribly swollen and touched the
floor as he stood beside Chris. Carefully I knelt down and
felt it. It was full of fluid. I rarely had anything to do with
dogs, and had certainly never seen anything like this before.
I didn't have an idea what it could be, although something
in the back of the lumber room of my memory seemed to
suggest it could be something to do with his heart.

'Look,' I admitted, 'dogs aren't really my territory. But
there's a new assistant at the practice on the small-animal
side who specializes in heart problems, and with Monty
being so old, there's a chance it could be that. And if anyone
can sort it out, Nick can. I think you should bring him in
tonight.'

Evening surgery started at 5.00 pm. Although I was in
early I noticed there was already a car in the car park, an only
too familiar Morris Minor Traveller, air-force grey trimmed
with varnished oak. As I went to check the next day's calls, I
glanced into the waiting room, and there she was, Miss
Heskins, with Horace in a wicker basket at her feet.

Horace was an extremely large ginger cat, adored by his
owner who, after the loss of both her brother and her fiancé
in the Battle of Britain, had no one else to lavish her
affection on. Miss Heskins was a wonderful old lady, but

she was one of nature's worriers. Horace rarely had anything much wrong with him in the conventional sense, but everything from the state of his claws to the wax in his ears was cause for Miss Heskins' alarm bells to go off. It was rare that a consultation with Horace lasted less than half an hour. The cat had been under the weather for about a month now, but I still hadn't been able to pinpoint exactly what was wrong and I was starting to dread the familiar cry, 'He's no better.'

Suddenly I had an idea and opened the door to the waiting room. Anyone watching would have spotted a wicked gleam in my eye. 'Miss Heskins,' I murmured, 'I wonder if I might have a word.'

Her face lit up. 'Oh, Mr Grant,' she said. 'That nice receptionist told me you would be doing surgery tonight so I came early to make sure not to miss you.'

'Well, Miss Heskins, it may turn out to be very good timing indeed. Since you were last here a new vet has joined the practice who, er,' I hesitated as I looked for the right word, 'specializes in cats. He's called Dr Lightfoot, and as luck would have it, he's here tonight.' Just then Nick put his head around the door.

'David, sorry to interrupt, but what's the SP on this dog that you want me to have a look at?'

As I followed him out, I nodded significantly towards Nick's disappearing back, and I noticed Miss Heskins do a little shuffle of anticipation on her seat.

I put Nick in the picture about Monty, as far as I could, and explained about Chris's emotional tie to the Labrador. It never ceased to puzzle me how a farmer could cheerfully send animals to market – and the small farmers I dealt with almost always knew their cows by name – and yet would mourn the death of a dog as if it were human.

I also asked Nick to look at Horace, saying that Horace was a puzzling case. As to Miss Heskins, I thought he would probably enjoy the consultation better if he had no warning.

Chris still hadn't arrived with Monty, so rather than keep Miss Heskins waiting any longer, Nick ushered her into Consulting Room No. 3. I was still in No. 4, the smallest, while Nick had gravitated to No. 3 with the partners always occupying 1 and 2 – there was a kind of hierarchy about it all.

Nick, who could quite legitimately be called Dr Lightfoot because of his PhD, was settling in well and the partners had lost no time in making use of his specialist knowledge. On a number of occasions I had seen him closeted with Peter and Frank, discussing some complicated investigation or diagnosis. To hear them was to get a glimpse of the high-tech world that small-animal practice was fast becoming. I had even started to feel left behind, having to remind myself that I would have time enough for small animals later. Meanwhile I was slowly picking up bits from the specialists whenever I spent any time in the consulting room.

Twenty-five minutes later I heard Miss Heskins' effusive thank-yous in the corridor. They had bonded – or rather Miss Heskins had – and I was off the hook.

Now that Nick was firmly ensconced as the small-animal specialist, my evening surgery was increasingly limited to routine vaccinations. One of my patients that evening was a black and white kitten belonging to a small girl who lived across the road from the hospital. Only a few weeks or so before a very similar-looking cat had been handed in, killed by one of the lorries that thundered past the surgery on their way to Dover. My suspicions were confirmed when her mother told me that her old cat Sooty had been run over and that Sweep was his replacement. How long would Sweep last, I wondered.

Nick collared me just as I was leaving.

'You were right, David. Interesting case.'

'Which one?' I countered.

'Oh the old Labrador. As for Horace, we'll just have to see when we get the results of the haematology, the old lady seems perfectly happy to foot the bill.'

'You have just met our best payer,' I laughed, and explained Miss Heskins' reputation for rapid settlement, not a trait we were familiar with on the farm side.

'No, it's the old dog that really interests me. You were right. Classic example of heart failure. Absolutely classic. Never seen an ascites quite so extreme though.' Ascites is the proper name for dropsy, where the heart can't pump blood around the body which results in it damming back, and fluid forming in the abdomen. 'Anyway, just thought I'd tell you. Nothing much I can do at the moment except put him on a diuretic and digoxin. But the owner, Chris whatshisname—'

'Oliver.'

'Yes. I mean, that's an old dog, David. But, just as you warned me, he was insistent that we did everything, so I've taken him in.'

The practice was not called a hospital for nothing. The former stables at the side of the big Edwardian house had been adapted as kennels for in-patients, with the two practice nurses who lived at the top of the house to keep an eye on them.

I had another night on call ahead of me but this time had no intention of going anywhere other than home for a quiet evening in with the telly and *Top Of The Pops*.

Chapter Three

Rumours were rife that the Beatles were about to split up and indeed they did a few months later. Everyone was splitting up. *Top of the Pops* began that night with Eric Clapton singing 'Comin' Home', his first solo single – Cream having split up earlier that year. Then it was downhill all the way; Johnny Cash singing 'A Boy Named Sue' and a children's TV performer called Rolf Harris singing 'Two Little Boys'. What had happened to rock 'n' roll? What had happened to the sixties?

What had happened was that they were all but over. It was November 1969. It wasn't long before Benny Hill made No. 1 with 'Ernie, the Fastest Milkman in the West'. The world was going mad, I decided. And I was growing old.

I was in bed by ten, which meant that when the phone rang at seven I had already had nearly ten hours' sleep. A farrowing. For once I had a leisurely shave and set off without bits of cotton wool stuck to my face where the razor had slipped.

As I put the car into gear I remembered that the first night call out I ever did on my own was a farrowing – the first I had ever done – at Paddy Dixon's when I ended up covered in mud and worse from head to toe and smelling like it for a week. I had no intention of that happening against this time. Nor was it likely. Pigs and I had developed a mutual respect that I, for one, took care never to abuse.

Still Practising

Most farrowings happen naturally, but sometimes there are just too many piglets and the sow gets tired. Once the process has started, if they aren't born quickly enough they die. Giving oxytocin makes the uterus contract more efficiently. I began idly to count up how many farrowings I'd done since I arrived. The early morning breakfast show was playing, appropriately enough an old Beatles classic, 'Here Comes the Sun', and I sang along as the Anglia gradually built up speed. The first time I had heard the Beatles was during my first term at college. It was 'Love Me Do' and their music had dominated my student years. I saw them only once, in Chatham, one of the three Medway towns, a few miles from Rochester. But the concerts I will never forget were those organized by our Student Union at Alexandra Palace in north London. One year we had the Rolling Stones and the whole college had to link arms to keep the fans off the stage. The next year was just as bad, with Donovan and the Who. They were having some trouble with the sound system and I will never forget Roger Daltrey strutting around the stage using some pretty ripe language – which fortunately the audience couldn't hear because the loudspeakers were down, but which I could hear every word of because I was so close. Then, when a roadie came out to tell him it was sorted, he roared out, 'That's class' and immediately went into the opening riff of 'My Generation'. It was a riot.

Four years on and I was in a different world. Another glorious day and this was my last night on call. Tonight Miss Caroline Hitchens was due at my 'gaff' as Keith called it. She was coming for supper and who knows what else: the house speciality of *chilli con carne* had been known to work wonders.

A straight stretch of road ribboned out before me but I

didn't put my foot down, preferring to enjoy the magic of driving into a Kentish sunrise. There wasn't a soul about, it was too early. Turner probably used Kentish sunrises for inspiration, I thought. Suddenly my bout of daydreaming came to an abrupt end when a policeman stepped out in front of me.

'Forty mile an hour limit on this road, sir. The signs are very clear. You've been clocked at fifty-two.'

I explained that I was a vet on call.

'Emergency, sir?' A combination of innate honesty and sheer stupidity made me blurt out, 'Well, no. Not really.'

Honestly was definitely not the best policy. A slow smile spread over the uniformed officer's face as he licked his pen and noted down the registration number of the car.

I couldn't believe what I had just said. All that education, a university degree, and my brain had come up with 'Well, no. Not really.' How thick can you get?

By now the copper was talking into a radio to his colleague half a mile up the road and in charge of the speed meter. I heard the walkie talkie crackled into life.

'Got a bloke 'ere says 'e's a vet. What's the drill Ken?'

Ken? Not Caroline's dad surely? It was worth a try.

'If that's Ken Hitchens, you might mention that his daughter Caroline and I are friends, in fact I'm seeing her tonight,' I added helpfully.

''E says to tell you that he's a friend of Caroline's.' Pause. Something unintelligible the other end. 'That's right, Ken. Caroline. Your Caroline. Seeing her tonight or something.'

Another pause, as the radio crackled into life again. He listened intently, nodding even more and then broke into an enormous grin.

'He says it's a first. You're nicked.'

Still Practising

When I arrived back at the practice, feeling as guilty as a schoolboy with a satchel full of scrumped apples, Frank was busy stitching up a kitten that had been attacked by a rabbit. He motioned me to come in. 'Bad news?'

I nodded. 'Sorry, Frank. Speeding.'

The senior partner sighed, pushed his glasses back over the bridge of his nose and carried on stitching the still body of the tabby kitten laid out on the operating table in front of him. 'What's that now?'

'How do you mean?'

'The tally, David. How many.'

'Two.'

'What happened about that red light business?'

'Nothing. They dropped the charges.'

A few weeks before I had gone through a red light at three in the morning and had been spotted by a bobby on the beat, who recognized the car.

'You must realize David, a vet without a licence is a vet without a job.'

I knew only too well. By now the rabbit that caused the kitten to need an operation was itself on the table, soon to be an ex-male. Castration was the only way to limit Flopsy's territorial instincts. Rabbits may look like cuddly toys, but once roused – by a playful kitten for example – their claws can do terrible damage. They're far tougher than a cat's: designed for digging rather than just tearing into flesh. In this case gashes to the kitten's face and hind-quarters needed thirteen stitches, whereas only two were needed to put paid to Flopsy's chances of becoming a daddy. Meanwhile the interrogation continued.

'How fast?'

Fifty-two they said.'

'Hmmm. Emergency?'

'Not really.' No need to go into unnecessary details, I decided.

Just then Nick's face appeared in the window, sparing me any further quizzing. Frank motioned him in.

'Sorry to interrupt, Frank, but I've got a bit of a problem.'

'Fire away.'

'There's this spaniel. And I just can't work out what's wrong. Looks perfectly healthy, just isn't eating. Everything's normal, temperature, pulse, respiration, heart, lungs. Generally not herself.'

'False pregnancy.' Frank and I couldn't have got it more together if we had rehearsed. As Nick was going through his textbook examination, the diagnosis had dawned on us both at precisely the same time. The moment Nick had said 'herself', my memory had flashed back to my first ever consultation when, faced with my first ever real unwell dog and a woman who couldn't stop crying, I began to wonder if I hadn't made a really bad career choice.

Nick looked from one to the other in amazement.

'Over to you,' said Frank, pointing the needle he was holding in my direction.

'You'll need to check and see if she has any milk,' I said. 'And find out when she was last in season.'

'Clever bastard, aren't you Grant,' Nick said later that afternoon as we made our way to the Spotted Cow for the traditional post-surgery pint.

'It's just experience, Lightfoot. Something you don't have much of,' then I ducked to avoid the inevitable cuff.

Canterbury must have more pubs than any other place of the same size. After Archbishop Thomas à Becket was murdered in the cathedral, the city became a place of pilgrimage. And even pilgrims needed somewhere to eat and drink and somewhere to stay. I had tried most of them, but always came back to the same two or three. The practice had the telephone numbers up on the notice board by reception, although I always told them where I could be reached when I was on call. The Spotted Cow was the nearest to the practice and had a garden, which was nice in summer.

There was no garden at the Olive Tree, where I had arranged to meet Caroline, as it was right in the centre of town, just outside the cathedral precincts. This place really was old. Unlike some of the pubs which, even in the late sixties had already started the business of 'knocking through' to make more space, the Olive Tree was a series of small interconnecting rooms where Chaucer himself could well have sat quaffing ale, let alone Dickens.

After a couple of pints I finally plucked up the courage to tell Caroline what had happened. She nearly choked on her crisps, roared with laughter, and proceeded to tell Jack, the landlord, who decided it was such a good story he would tell the rest of his customers. Eventually, even I had to laugh – although it wouldn't seem so funny when I got the summons.

A week or so later Caroline invited me to Sunday lunch and I finally got to meet her father properly. He turned out to be a great family man, but I never quite got used to the idea of him being a copper. We ended up talking about birds; he was a great bird watcher and used to spend hours down at the marshes watching waterfowl. I didn't contest the speeding, so Sergeant Hitchens did not have to give evidence against me. Now that wouldn't have been pleasant.

Back at the hospital life continued as usual. As far as Horace the ginger cat was concerned, Nick had decided that a more detailed investigation was required and admitted him for a complete 'work-up', a phrase which had just appeared in the American literature, and which meant that every possible test would be done.

A week or so later I heard him discussing the results with Miss Heskins. All the routine haematology had come back normal. There was no evidence of liver or kidney disease – in fact there was no evidence of anything at all. 'We shall opt for scientific observation,' I overheard Nick saying loftily, 'and see if anything develops. In the meantime I will give him a pick-me-up injection.'

I glanced through the door and saw him drawing up a vitamin B12 injection. It was a lovely purple colour and looked the part for curing an ailing moggie, although it was doubtful that it would make the slightest bit of difference to whatever was wrong with Horace.

The expression on Miss Heskins' face wavered between relief and concern. Nick noticed and responded just as I thought he would. Just as I had done in fact. 'And if you're worried – don't hesitate to give us a call.'

I tried to stifle a laugh. Hearing me, Nick swivelled on his chair, by which time I had managed to turn it into a cough, waved my hand to Miss Heskins and scurried to back to Consulting Room 4.

Miss Heskins was justly famous for her late night calls. I thought about warning Nick to go to bed early the next time he was on duty but he pre-empted me five minutes later by inviting me round for dinner that evening. 'I'm on duty,' he explained, 'so I can drop you off afterwards.'

As the alternative was a steak pie from the local fish and chip shop, I didn't need much persuading. I accepted the invitation and nipped home to change while Nick was seeing the last client of the day.

Still Practising

While Selina was busying herself in the kitchen, Nick and I talked shop by the open fire. It was only a small grate but, like many in these old Victorian houses, it pumped out a fair volume of heat.

Monty, Chris Oliver's old dog, hadn't responded to the drugs at all. All Nick could do was to drain his abdomen of the fluid manually by sticking a 16-gauge needle in his stomach, just like the needle used for milk fever in a cow and wait until the fluid came out. Then his skin would pull back and he would look like a normal dog again. But it didn't last long, because the heart wasn't pumping properly, and so every two or three weeks Chris and Monty would be back. It was time consuming and expensive for a small farmer living over half an hour away. Each session took a good forty-five minutes, but there was no question of putting Monty down.

As it turned out he lived another six months and just died in his sleep. In the thirty years since then there have been such advances in drug development that the draining wouldn't have been necessary at all. But there was a positive outcome: after six months of this time-consuming procedure, Chris and Nick had spent hours talking and had become firm friends. It turned out that they were both steam and sailing fanatics, two things that I have never been able to get worked up about.

As I had anticipated, Selina did us proud. The first course was a creamy cheese tart – what I soon learned was called a quiche, then something quite new. The pastry bore no resemblance to the pastry my mother used to make, or that I had at Peggoty's Pantry for that matter, but crumbled at the touch of a fork and practically dissolved in the mouth. This time it was Nick who was off the booze while I was happily enjoying a French wine from the Loire valley that was to become a favourite, Sancerre.

'Well, apart from that emergency with you the other week, the night duties so far have been a piece of cake,' announced the veteran of less than a month who, as far as I could judge, had hardly been out of Canterbury.

He had forgotten the first rule of night duty. Don't tempt fate. As if in answer, the phone rang. Selina answered and passed it to Nick, giving me a look and raising her eyebrows.

'Yes, Frank. Er, no Frank, can't say I have. But wait a minute, David's here.' He turned towards me, an agonized look on his face, and mouthed something I could not make head or tail of. I hunched my shoulders. Obviously an emergency. Nick, put the phone down. He looked as white as a sheet.

'Bloat,' he said, 'a cow with bloat.' It turned out that Charles Harte, the other farm-animal partner on call, was out on the marshes with a difficult calving.

Although I had been qualified for nearly two years, I had never come across bloat, though I knew a good deal about it. Like any other cinemagoer I had seen it portrayed in sheep in a famous scene in *Far from the Madding Crowd*. This was as good a time as any to gain practical experience I decided, and Selina said that our main course could wait.

There are two types – simple bloat and frothy bloat – and a myriad of causes, including eating grass that is too fresh. For whatever reason gas is produced in the abdomen that the cow can't get rid of in the usual way. They say now that the methane that cows discharge into the air through flatulence destroys the ozone layer with greater efficiency than vehicle pollution.

What we would have to do was pass a stomach tube into the cow and give her the anti-bloat drench, a mixture of vegetable oils, or in the worst scenario plunge a trocar and canula – which looks like a medieval instrument of torture

– into the stomach. This was a devilish looking thing which was basically a sharp dagger surrounding a tube. The dagger went in and left the tube in the stomach, and the trapped gas would escape.

I checked in Nick's boot for the trocar and canula and made sure we had local anaesthetic and stitch up materials and then we set off. This was the first time I had driven with Nick and I felt like a navigator in a rally car as we sped down country lanes with me shouting directions. The arc of mud he had shot up when we had left Roy Gibbons' place that first night was no slip of the accelerator. It turned out that he really was a rally driver – it was one of his many hobbies. He headed into every bend at a speed that made me think we would never get round it, braked, changed down, then it was foot down again, change up and away. I had reckoned on twenty minutes, but within fifteen minutes we were there – and in the nick of time.

I had heard of Major Boyce, as he was always called, but never been to his farm. He had a reputation for being difficult. Invalided out of the army with a burst eardrum, he had never lost the manner or the doing-it-by-book attitude. Improvization was not a concept he understood. Charles was the only one he seemed to get on with, and so Charles it always was who went to see him.

'Two of you,' he barked, as we both jumped out of the car. 'I hope this doesn't mean I'll be charged double.' This was becoming something of a running joke, but on this occasion it was said without any humour. The major was already marching towards the far side of the yard, where the patient was by now lying flat out, gasping for breath. Her whole side was ballooned out and as tight as a drum. First I opened her mouth: the colour of her gums was dreadful, a mixture of grey and purple. She was obviously on her last

David Grant

legs – it was too late for stomach tubes and anti-bloat drench.

I found a blade and made a nick in the skin at its highest point over the massive swelling on her side. Then, taking a deep breath I plunged the trocar in. A huge gush of gas came out and the swelling went down in front of our eyes. Nick and I looked at each other in triumph. Then I glanced back at the major and realized with horror that he had put a pipe in his mouth and with shaking hands was about to light a match.

'Don't!' I shouted. 'You'll cause an explosion!'

The gas trapped in the cow's rumen was pure methane – the cause of many a pit disaster in the past as it was so inflammable.

The man was clearly shaken and leaned for support against the fence.

Nick then stitched the canula into the skin so that for the time being there would be a permanent outlet for any further gas, and I arranged to visit the next morning. We could then investigate what had caused it to try and prevent this happening again. I made a mental note to talk to Alan and take *Merck's Veterinary Manual* to work with me.

It was nearly ten by the time we get back to Canterbury. Selina was busy on the floor sorting sheets of coloured paper ready for her class the next day. Who says a teacher's work is finished when the bell rings?

Although the quiche had kept us going, we were both ready for the next course. It seemed only minutes before a plate heaped with ribbon noodles and a creamy mixture of meat and chopped spring onions was in front of us. Beef stroganoff apparently. I took a hungry mouthful, and gave a groan of pleasure. The meat was the most tender I have ever tasted.

'Fillet steak,' said Nick proudly.

I was suitably impressed. Fillet steak was always the most expensive on the menu.

'But the best trick is that Selina buys the tail of fillet, which butchers round here sell cheap; they don't know what to do with it.'

'It should be made with sour cream,' explained Selina, 'but I can't find any in Canterbury. Silly isn't it? With all these cows, they must have made it in the old days. So I just add lemon juice to ordinary cream.'

Then came a green salad. This was all so new. Salad had always meant something involving half a tomato and a piece of beetroot and a few lettuce leaves. This was a tumble of lettuce, spinach and, believe it or not, dandelion leaves.

'You know there are so many things out there we can eat, that people have always eaten for hundreds of years. Thousands even. It's a real waste, and I'm going to do some research into it at the local library. You won't mind being my guinea pig, will you David?' she added, her eyes glinting impishly.

'Not if the results are as good as this,' I said as I followed Nick's example, wiping my plate with a piece of bread to soak up the salad dressing. Why had I never done this before? Probably because it's just not the same with salad cream.

'But before that I want to see an animal being born. I think it will make me understand more, feel more part of the place. What do you think, David?'

I nodded, too contented to speak. Was this what marriage is all about I wondered? Wonderful food and a woman who's interested in what you do, and yet who has a life of her own? I decided to turn down Nick's offer of a lift and walked home. Nick came with me to the end of the street. It was a beautiful night – there wouldn't be many more of them before the wind straight off the North Sea, which can make Kent feel as cold as the Scottish moors, got a grip. Canterbury is only a few miles from the sea in any direction, and during the day the sound of seagulls is never far away in case you need reminding.

'Night duties aren't that bad,' Nick said as he turned back towards the house. 'You've been exaggerating! I should learn to take everything you say with a pinch of salt.'

'Nick, when will you learn, don't tempt fate.'

The fates were obviously listening, because next morning Nick's cheerful face of the previous night had been totally extinguished. I caught sight of him in Consulting Room 3 trying to keep a guinea pig from falling off the table. He looked completely clapped out. Jackie, the junior practice nurse, told me that he had been called out to Rupert Charlton-Jones' place. The family had been to a hunt ball and arrived back at two in the morning to find a cow calving.

Nick and Selina were soundly asleep by the time the phone call came, and of course it woke Selina as well. This was her chance to witness a calf being born! But by the time they got there, it was too late – nature had already taken its course. But the sight of the tiny calf was enough for Selina – until the next time anyway. Then just as Nick was dropping off to sleep, the phone went again. It was Charles. Could Nick phone Miss Heskins. There had been a development apparently with Horace.

Not wanting to wake Selina who was by then sound asleep he went downstairs to make the call. Miss Heskins, he later told me, had sounded as bright as a button. 'Oh Dr Lightfoot. I'm so pleased you got my message. I know you have been just as worried as I have about Horace. I haven't slept properly for weeks you know. Well, Horace was asleep on the foot of my bed as usual, and then there was this dreadful noise. I really thought he was going to die. He seemed to be in terrible pain, his poor body contorting. I didn't know what to do. And then it happened.'

'What happened, Miss Heskins?'

'The grey thing. It was the size of a mouse. A large grey mouse, but no legs and more sausage-shaped. And ever since then, he's been quite his old self. I didn't call earlier as I felt I should wait until I was sure.'

'That was very thoughtful of you, Miss Heskins.'

'Will you want to do an autopsy on it?'

'A what, Miss Heskins?'

'An autopsy, test, whatever-you-call it, on the grey thing.'

'Well, next time you're passing Miss Heskins. But I shouldn't worry too much.'

Nick recounted the conversation later that evening in the Spotted Cow. Horace's mystery illness was, of course, a fur ball, admittedly a large one. And the idea of us doing a biopsy on a matted collection of Horace's lickings had us all in fits of laughter.

I had slept soundly until the alarm went off at eight – a full seven hours – and I was feeling on top of the world. The sight of Nick's still rumpled face reminded me how the tables had turned. Better still, while I was enjoying a pint of Kent's finest ale, Shepherd Neame bitter, Nick was nursing an orange juice mixed with soda water. Last night had been just the first of his five-nights on the trot stint.

Chapter Four

When I was a child the countryside was somewhere for bicycle rides with my father. Rochester, where I was born and brought up, stands where the River Medway joins the Thames. It's really the Medway rising in the South Downs and meandering its way north across the Weald that makes Kent one of the most fertile regions in England.

Five minutes out of Rochester and we were deep in the heart of the countryside. Since I was eight or nine hardly a Sunday had passed without Dad and me setting out on our racers. Before the war he had been a champion cyclist. He built the bikes himself, and even when I had left home he still kept mine oiled and ready for use. Cycling is the most strenuous exercise there is, which meant that by the time I started running competitively I had a head start on my rivals. I was super fit, though never as energy efficient as Dad.

Our route always began the same way: through the village of Borstal, where the idea of separate educational prisons for young offenders first started, then the climb up Bluebell Hill, the escarpment that rises to the south of Rochester. It was always a real push but what an amazing view when you got there. To a young boy like me, it felt as though the whole world was spread out below us. At the top was a café and we'd stop and have a cup of coffee and a marshmallow before pushing on. I still remember those marshmallows.

Still Practising

My dad continued cycling well into his seventies. And whenever I went home, out would come the bikes and it would be just like the old days, though in later years it wasn't the promise of marshmallows that got me to the top of Bluebell Hill, but a pint. Even if I hadn't been home for months, my bike would always be there in the shed ready for me, in tip top condition. The ritual was always the same. We would take it gently till we got to the top of Bluebell Hill then, after a short pause to admire the view, we mounted up again and pedalled like bats out of hell along the single track that ran across the ridge to the pub. It was never anything less than a life and death contest between us, because the loser paid. The last time we did this, Dad was seventy. I jumped him at the start and went flat out but about 50 yards from the pub there was a flash of dust as he drew parallel then, head low over the handlebars, he took me. The canny old man had been in my slip stream all the way, waited till he saw me falter, then went for it. Nine years later he died of lung cancer. He'd always been so fit, never a day's illness, but he'd been a smoker all his life and when he started in the thirties nobody knew what it did to you. I was lucky. Even when I was young everyone knew that it wasn't something you should do if you were an athlete, so I've never smoked.

When I was growing up, there didn't seem to be a thing that my dad didn't know. Every question had its answer. On those cycle rides I learned to identify everything we passed, from birds of prey hovering above the stubble in the early spring to the orchards of apples, pears, plums and cherries that bordered our favourite route, the Pilgrims' Way. In the autumn there were blackberries and hazelnuts to collect, or sometimes filberts, a fat variety of hazelnut that my mother was very partial to. I have never lost my love of the country

David Grant

and I owe that to the good grounding I got from my dad.

The orchards and nut groves were often planted in grid-like precision, and the trees were usually much smaller than you would get in a garden, no higher than a man's shoulder, to make picking easier. Hop gardens looked to me like an impenetrable jungle such as you might find in the Amazon, all twisting vines that by midsummer were nearly strangling each other, followed by the sad sight in late September of row upon row of empty canes and wires stretching between them, sagging now but still carrying odd pieces of vine.

I didn't know then what pleasure the hops could bring, but just a few years later I became a small part of the process of beer-making. Although I had a student grant – and without it I could never have become a vet – it never went far enough and every September I worked on the Guinness hop farm outside Faversham. My job was to drive the tractor in between the hop vines. The tractor had a platform above it where six or so women would stand, picking the ripe hops. Although I couldn't see them, I could certainly hear them and blushed at the ripe Cockney language, most of which I knew was for my benefit. The work was hard. I set off from Rochester at 7.30 in a 1940 Morris convertible that Dad had bought for £30. Most days I drove with the top down. I loved that car and can still remember the number: COW 881, very appropriate for a trainee vet.

We worked through until 6.00 p.m. with forty-five minutes for lunch, a slice of bread 2 inches thick and a slab of cheese not much smaller at a pub called the Ploughman washed down with a pint of Shepherd Neame. The women came too and never stopped ragging me because I was a student. I remember there was one young girl about my age whom I tried to chat up. It came as quite a shock when she told me that she thought I wouldn't want to talk to someone like her. Just the fact that I was a student set me apart, although I was only a working-class lad myself. These women were all from London's East End and came back year after year. Although it was backbreaking work they treated it as a holiday. I did it every summer I was a student and grew to love the smell of the hops, a very bitter ripe smell.

Neither then nor when I was a boy had it ever occurred to me that farming was a hard life. In the evenings cycling home with my dad we would sometimes come across cows on their way to the farm be milked. But there never seemed to be a rush about it. The farmer would be wandering behind these great beasts with his collie dog and unfailingly gave me and my dad a cheery wave. And of course in my rose-tinted memory, it was always summer, and always sunny.

But now that I was a cog in the farming wheel, I soon learned that this picture postcard view of country life was a long way from reality. The farmers I met might own their land (although many didn't), but profit margins on livestock-rearing or dairy farms were tight. The cows had to be milked twice a day, every day, including Christmas. First milking was often at five in the morning, with the milker having to get up even earlier to get the cows in to the parlour. There are innumerable hard jobs around the farm to do and mostly these were done by men, although occasionally I came across women who did just as much.

Janet Potter was one such. Her mother and father had farmed for years but by the time I met them they were getting on and it was Janet, in her early thirties, who did the lion's share of the milking and general running of the farm. The Potters did a bit of everything: cows, sheep and fruit. They didn't have any outside help, except for the cherry

51

harvest when they brought in a gang of pickers, although even then Janet was out with them from dawn till dusk at the backbreaking work.

Theirs had been one of the first farms I had visited with Alan Jenkins the day I started work at the practice – which already seemed like years ago. And what an introduction. It seemed idyllic, looking like something off a calendar, a farmhouse that once must have been rather grand, overhung by a copper beech tree hundreds of years old. Janet was small and slight, with a quiet, dignified manner. She didn't laugh a lot and took her job seriously. I'd never heard any talk of a man friend and, as far as I knew, she hadn't taken a holiday in years. Her main hobby and relaxation was oil painting, and it always surprised me when I caught sight of those tiny hands on her sturdy body covered in layers of shapeless clothes.

I always enjoyed going to the Potters' place. Not many people visited the farm, and although outwardly very quiet, I think Janet enjoyed the company. With a bit of persuasion she would always show me her latest work, but only if I asked. She was one of the most unassuming people I have ever met. Her paintings hung all over the house, and I enjoyed the opportunity of seeing beyond the kitchen. There was an intricate carved staircase and, to the right of a chimney breast in the hall a small wooden door, not much bigger than a telephone directory, that she told me was a wig cupboard. The complicated wigs that even quite ordinary people wore in the seventeenth and eighteenth centuries were very costly, she explained, and had to be kept away from damp and rats.

I hadn't been to see the Potters for several months, though I had heard that John Potter had spent a week in the local cottage hospital following a couple of small strokes.

Although he was back home now, I knew that Janet would make sure she bore the brunt of the work. And I was not mistaken. But it was still odd to think that the diminutive figure shifting a large bale of corn and then manhandling a even larger beast into the stockade for my benefit was the same person who could capture the translucence of a wood anemone in oil paint.

She needed to get the animal boxed in so that I could look at its feet. It had the usual 'foul in the foot' – another of these fantastic terms which hung on from almost medieval times. It was an infection caused by a germ, and with modern antibiotics was relatively easy to treat. The first thing to do is to trim back the diseased hoof to let the poison out, then follow this up with a jab of penicillin. The cow doesn't like it but with you holding one of her feet there's not a lot she can do to object.

Although it was only November the main thing on Janet's mind that morning was her sheep. I had noticed that most of her ewes were marked at the rear with a telltale blue dye, proof that the ram had done his stuff and they were 'in tup'. When the ram is put to the ewes a small box of blue dye is strapped to his chest so that when he mounts the ewe – which she'll only let him do when she's in season – she gets marked.

The Potters' flock ran to a couple of hundred and they always put their ewes to the ram early because there was a better price for Easter lamb. Early lambing might be more lucrative but it is also more dangerous than spring lambing. Even so, I had never been called out to a lambing at the Potters. Janet had very small hands and these could deftly remove a lamb whenever a ewe was having difficulty giving birth without causing suffering. And if a mother rejected her offspring or died – as did sometimes happen if the

labour was very stressful – then Janet, like many farmers'
womenfolk down the years, would take on the job of bottle-
feeding the lamb with watered-down cow's milk, a time-
consuming business. Lambs need feeding even more
regularly than human babies – once every two hours,
twenty-four-hours a day. Hand-reared lambs usually
attached themselves to their human 'mother' and it was
hard to resist these fluffy creatures, flopping around the
kitchen, like family pets. But there was no room for senti-
mentality in a working farm, and only rarely did I hear of
such orphans being spared the fate of their brothers and
sisters.

Work over, Janet took me through into their simple
sitting room to see some of her recent work, mainly land-
scapes with some views of the old buildings in town. As I
looked at them, I was surprised to see a price sticker. Oh
yes, she told me. They were for sale. She exhibited them in
country fairs and local galleries.

'Not the sort of places I generally go,' I admitted as I
alternately stood back to admire them, then went closer to
look at the detail. The one with the price on was a beautiful
picture of a spring woodland.

'I didn't finish that one until the summer,' explained
Janet. 'And people generally like to buy one that captures
the season they're in, so it didn't sell. But it will next
spring.'

I was no better. The pictures that had caught my eye
were all painted in the rich browns and russets capturing to
perfection the autumn Kentish scenery that lay all around.
There was one in particular that struck me. It showed an old
bridge over a stream, and in the foreground beech trees
dipped down towards the water and their rich russet leaves
were reflected in the water. It wasn't too big, about the size

of a poster. Janet told me the stream was a branch of the Stour, about 3 miles from the house. There was just a track over the bridge which was a public bridleway. The picture had no frame, just the canvas wrapped around the stretchers. I could just see it on the wall above my settee.

'How much is this one?'

'Oh,' she said, somewhat taken aback. 'Don't feel you have to buy anything, David.'

'Come on, Janet. How much?' I repeated.

'Ten pounds.'

That was easily within my reach. I had had a couple of weekends on duty in quick succession and quite a few nights during the week. I hadn't been able to get out and spend my hard-earned cash even if I had wanted to. I thought it might be nice to see where it was painted and Janet got out an old Ordnance Survey map to show me. I might go there with Caroline, I thought. There was a pub I'd heard was quite good a couple of miles away. We could make a day of it. Caroline hadn't been back to Canterbury for several weeks and wouldn't be now till Christmas. Buying the picture seemed to have the effect of an adrenalin rush, and before I knew it I had bought two more, one which I planned to give my mother, and another just because I liked it.

As I left I carefully loaded three paintings into the back seat of the Anglia £30 worse off – a week and a half's wages – but with paintings that still hang in my mother's house thirty years later. Also in the boot was a bottle of Mrs Potter's elderberry wine, an early Christmas present she said. Judging by the old lady's smile I knew the money was a welcome addition to the tight finances of the farm. As I left Janet was already busy calling the cows in from the fields for the second session of milking – it would be hours before she could call it a day and even then she would be on her late rounds before turning in. Those late rounds were done by all the farmers – and were the source of many a late-night call if they found anything amiss.

'All ready for tonight, then? 7.30. Don't be late.' Nick tapped his watch as he disappeared into Consulting Room No. 3. 'Believe me, you're in for a treat, you uncultured slob.'

Selina's friend Kiki was appearing at the Marlowe Theatre and Nick had said I could hardly go there for supper and not see the play. The theatre was right in the old part of town. It had once been a cinema and, although it looked older than it was, had presumably been something else before that. I had often passed it but had never been in. It was named after the Elizabethan playwright Christopher Marlowe, who was born in Canterbury but whom I had never heard of before I read the programme. The play was *The Servant of Two Masters* by Carlo Goldoni. Although I had been to see Shakespeare with my school, this was the first time I could remember going to the theatre out of choice. But when Nick had shown me the publicity poster, there was no stopping me.

Nick was right. I wasn't disappointed. The play was very funny, particularly one scene I remember that involved the servant serving supper to both his masters. He was starving and he did it very convincingly – just watching him made me hungry. Selina had warned me not to eat beforehand, as she had prepared something special.

The play was set in the eighteenth century and the three female characters all had precocious amounts of bosom showing, laced and squeezed into costumes that were barely big enough. When the actresses did their curtsies at the end of the play, they bent right forward. We were right at the front and I was convinced something was going to fall out. I said as much to Nick in the pub as we waited for the girls – Selina had gone up to see her friend in the dressing room.

'It's all held in with Sellotape,' he volunteered.

Just at that moment they came in. If it hadn't been for the hour-glass figure, I would hardly have recognized Kiki as the same person up on stage. I realized she had been wearing a wig. Her own hair was short, cut in a spiky, elfin style. Her eyes were still covered in eye shadow and mascara but the rest of her face was bare.

'It's all done with Sellotape, isn't it, Kiki?' said Nick as he pulled out a chair for her.

'What is, darling?'

'Your boobs.'

'Of course, I told you that the other night.'

'Yes, but David here didn't believe me, did you?'

All eyes swivelled in my direction and not for the first time with the Lightfoots I was completely wrong-footed and lost for words.

'Take any notice of him,' said Kiki and flashed me a smile that, if you could plug it in to the national grid, would save a fortune.

'To listen to Nick you'd think it was some kind of kinky perversion,' she continued. 'The Sellotape is just instead of a bra. You can't wear one you see because it would show, so we just use Sellotape instead.'

It was clear I had to say something.

'Doesn't it hurt,' I ventured, finally having found my voice; 'er – pulling it off?'

'Oh yes, but, then what doesn't, darling?' And she flashed me another of those smiles.

Of course I had often heard that actors and actresses

David Grant

called each other darling, but as I had never met one before, I had never really believed it happened in real life and I certainly hadn't realized it applied to people who weren't actors, like me. But Kiki said it quite naturally. So who was I to complain?

By the time we left the pub, it was gone eleven and I was starving. A bottle of wine was soon opened and we sat down to eat. We began with a dish I did not recognize at all. Not that that was saying much. Circles of something or other in a dark syrupy sauce.

'Cheers, everybody,' Nick raised his glass. 'And well done Kiki. Smashing show, really enjoyed it.'

Kiki, who had gone upstairs to change out of the jeans and jumper she had come to the pub in, had returned looking stunning in a short skirt and low-cut top that didn't cover up much more than the costume. I wondered what they had said about me: sad bloke who hasn't got a bird, or sexy bloke who is a real catch?

'So. Tuck in everybody, don't wait,' said Selina.

'What is it?' I asked as I tried to get one of these things on my fork. There was a moment's pause when Selina looked at Nick, and then he spoke.

'Bollocks.'

My fork froze in my hand. 'What?'

'Bollocks,' he repeated, 'Bullocks' bollocks. Or if you'd rather, bullocks' testicles. Cooked in Madeira weren't they, darling?'

Testicles! The very thought was painful. To think I had nearly eaten them.

'Ummmm,' he said, as he took another mouthful. 'Absolutely delicious, hun. Nothing like eating something that hasn't cost you anything. I must ask Alan to get me some more the next time he does a big castration.'

Still Practising

Alan had given them to him? I just couldn't believe it. I knew he had done a big castration job that morning, but surely . . .

'What do you think Kiki? Good aren't they.'

'Dee – li – shus,' she enunciated. 'Can only vets get them or do you think my butcher in the King's Road could find some for me?'

'I doubt that very much because they're not from dead animals you see. The chaps these balls belonged to are still in fine fettle, aren't they David?'

Something had happened to my stomach. Although a few minutes ago I had been ravenously hungry, now I felt something remarkably like nausea. I pushed my plate away.

'What?' said Nick. 'Not hungry David?'

I don't know who started laughing first. I think it was Selina. But very soon they all had tears rolling down their faces.

'It was a joke, David,' Selina eventually managed to splutter. 'A joke. They're not testicles at all, just squid, octopus.' At which they all collapsed in another fit of laughter.

If Selina imagined that the idea of eating octopus was any better, she was mistaken. And, to be frank, I have never really been happy with squid since. It was Kiki who came to my rescue.

'I think they're being perfectly horrid to you,' she said. 'I think what you need is a bit of cheering up. Because I like you.' She went across to the record player and the next minute I was dancing with this gorgeous woman to Elvis Presley singing 'The Wonder Of You'. I had never been an Elvis fan before, but for some reason I began to warm to him.

By now all the laughter had died away. Selina and Nick

cleared away the plates and by the time the last strains of Elvis had died away and I had reluctantly let my dancing partner go, I could smell roast chicken which was, as usual, delicious. My appetite had returned.

'You will forgive me, won't you, David?' Selina said later as I helped clear the table. 'But you were so keen to try everything that when I remembered Nick telling me about some students he knew who had eaten testicles, I just couldn't resist it. You mustn't blame Nick, it was me.'

'I forgive you,' I said.

'Anyway,' Selina added under her breath. 'It certainly brought you close to a certain person. I think you've made a hit there.'

Kiki was only in Canterbury for a week. And Caroline was away in London. I looked over at the impish face and amazing body as she gave me a wink. With a start I realized that I didn't feel a trace of guilt about what might happen.

Chapter Five

Shortly before Christmas I was just getting out of the car back at the practice when Alan called me. He was sporting a fine spray of winter jasmine in his buttonhole and had someone I didn't know standing beside him. It was very cold. We stood with our hands in our pockets, our breath freezing in the air as we spoke.

'Ah David. Just the chap,' he said clapping me on the back. 'Want you to meet Duncan. I think Frank might have mentioned him to you. Duncan will be seeing practice for a month or so.' He looked at his watch.

'Look,' he said, 'I'd been hoping to take Duncan for lunch but I've got a sick goat who won't wait, so must dash. Think you could do the honours for me? Then take him on your rounds with you, show him the ropes. You're off to Paddy Dixon's for a vaccination follow-up I think. And there's a horse we've just had a call about from the Armistead place. Same direction, so perhaps you could drop in and have a look-see will you? Pauline will give you the details. Doesn't sound too urgent. Horse off his food.'

The sky had turned battleship grey, and it was trying to snow. I knew we'd be hard pushed to get anything to eat on a Monday at a country pub and I didn't fancy taking him to Peggoty's Pantry; I'd be sure to get a barrage of questions from Joan about Caroline and I didn't want to have to explain everything to a complete stranger. So we ended up going where we so often ended up going, the Spotted Cow,

David Grant

where at least I could rely on Theo the landlord to have the log fire in the inglenook blazing away and a sandwich or a meat pie and chips.

Any thoughts I'd entertained that this new student would be a good laugh were swiftly dispelled. Duncan came from Selkirk in the Scottish Borders. He didn't drink. He wasn't interested in sport or women. All Duncan was interested in was Duncan and Duncan's future career. As a fourth-year student he could only have been twenty-one or perhaps twenty-two, but his attitude to life was like a 45-year-old's. But even saying that I am maligning most 45-year-olds. As for his dress sense, he made me seem like George Best. He wore the kind of clothes your mother might have bought when you were fourteen, hoping that you would grow into them. Not that this was very uncommon among veterinary students at the time, who – if they weren't as mad as hatters – might easily be mistaken for Theology students. Nick, Frank and Alan – and I like to think myself – fell into the mad-as-hatters category. Only Charles Harte among the partners belonged to the other strain.

Paddy Dixon's piglets were all doing well and 'his girls' were coping with their enormous litters without any problems. The yard was very icy and where the sun hadn't reached, puddles in the mud crunched underfoot. But when we sat down for the usual cup of tea made by Eileen, Duncan launched into the nearest thing to an interrogation outside the X-Ray room, where Nick and I were still regularly summoned when we'd strayed from the path of good practice.

What did Paddy feed his weaners on? Wasn't that too strong? What prophylactic drugs did he give them? How did he gauge the amounts? How many pigs to the square yard? And on and on it went, with Duncan demanding the kind of statistics that were to become the bane of farmers' lives when Britain eventually became part of the Common Market. At one point Paddy went to refill the kettle and, standing behind Duncan, gave me a look as if to say, 'Am I mad, or is he mad?' It was all I could do not to start laughing.

When Eileen offered us both another scone, I had to refuse. I had always enjoyed the time I spent with the Dixons, but this time I knew I had to get away as soon as possible. I explained that there was a horse to see a few miles away, collected my kit and after hosing our waders down with the usual mix of water and disinfectant, set off again.

Most of my clients were working farmers, some richer, some poorer, but Sir John Armistead was a justice of the peace whose family had lived at Merriston Place for centuries and was, I imagined, richer than all the practice's other clients put together. I had passed the entrance, two eighteenth-century gatehouses, many times, but I had never seen the house, which I discovered was nearly a mile from the road. The drive wound down through typical English parkland dotted with trees that, in the grey winter light looked like a drawing by an old master. Everything was eerily quiet. Nothing moved. There was frost still on the north side of the hills and mist was beginning to form in the hollows.

Like the gatehouses, the house was built not of the local brick but of limestone. It was huge, like something out of Jane Austen. The wings on either side of the main house were lined with pillars. On a ridge to our left the remains of a building jutted out against the sky – some kind of old castle. The Anglia felt decidedly out of place.

David Grant

Pauline, the practice secretary, had said we should go round the back. But where was the back? The car crunched to a standstill on the gravel forecourt to one side of the main portico. To his obvious annoyance I told Duncan to stay in the car while I found out where we had to go. Would they have something as mundane as a bell, I wondered? Or should I go to the tradesman's entrance? I would have done if I'd known where it was. I discovered later than the tradesman's entrance was round the other side, as tradesmen came on a different road from an entirely different direction, completely hidden from the house, so that visitors and family would not have to witness their comings and goings. Tentatively I rang an iron bell set in the stonework beside the front door that was the size of a garage door. But it made no sound at all. I had just turned away when one half swung open.

I had expected a butler but it was a young woman in jeans with a small child balanced on her hip.

'Good afternoon,' I began. 'I was looking for Lady Armistead. It's about her horse. I'm the vet.'

'Oh come in. I'm the nanny. The children are just having tea, come through.'

The hall was the size of half a tennis court. The floor was a chequerboard of black and white marble and the heels of my shoes, which had recently been mended with a metal strip, made enough noise to waken the dead. Behind the hall was a corridor which seemed to run the width of the house. We turned right, then took another corridor to the left until finally we came to an open door that led into an amazing room, 40 feet long at least, with three sets of French windows opening onto a terrace, and beyond the terrace you could see the lake settling into the dusk.

On the floor in front of a roaring fire set 2 feet up in the wall, were two small children hitting wooden shapes through holes in a board with what I imagine was a rubber hammer. On a large settee beside them sat a girl wearing black leather trousers, high boots and a fringed silk top weighed down with necklaces. As we came in, she turned and flashed me a friendly smile.

'It's the vet, Dodie.'

Dodie? And it was only then that I remembered and, of course, recognized the smile. Dodie Mason had been one of the faces of the sixties. It was soon after I had started college that Sir John Armistead, whose wife had been killed falling off a horse, had married the 18-year-old model. It had caused quite a scandal at the time because the new bride was younger than Sir John's youngest son. I hadn't heard anything of either of them since.

'Mr Grant, isn't it?' Her voice was a surprise, much lower and softer than I expected. I had imagined she might have had a grating, Eliza Doolittle kind of voice, but it was quite husky.

'Er, yes. David Grant.' To say I was flustered was an understatement.

'Thanks for coming out. I know I'm probably being very silly, but I'm worried about Seamus. He's so adorable. And I don't even know how to take his temperature!' her laugh was as soft and mesmerizing as the gurgle of a stream.

Seamus was a roan colt and over the last day or so had lost his 'spirit' as Dodie put it, and a few hours earlier he had had 'a bit of a turn'. Pauline hadn't mentioned anything about that – just stiff joints. When I asked her what she meant, the former model said she couldn't really explain. She didn't know much about horses, she said. I didn't like to tell her that I didn't either. She wondered if he could have arthritis because he seemed to be moving rather strangely, as if he were stiff.

The stables lay to the right of the main drive. To get there you left one world and entered another, literally through a door covered in green baize which made a soft thud as it closed. This was the servants' quarters. Separate stairs – much smaller than the grand staircase that I had seen in the black and white hall – went up to the next floor. Everything was much smaller and meaner except for the kitchen, which was as big as the room we had just been in, with a stone flagged floor and a huge table in the middle with a woman at the far end peeling potatoes, who I realized was the cook when they started discussing menus. She was a large woman who looked remarkably like Hattie Jacques. It was only then that I remembered Duncan. I excused myself and said I'd be back in a couple of minutes with my colleague.

Duncan was sitting in the car reading *Merck's Veterinary Manual* by the light of the large torch that I always carried with me in the glove compartment. I had excuses all prepared for having left him, but as he was all smiles when I arrived I decided to forget them.

'Well? What is it?'

'I don't know, Duncan. Haven't seen the patient yet.'

I changed into my waders – Duncan already had his on – and then we made our way around to the kitchen, but her ladyship had already gone to the stables, the cook informed me.

The whole scene was like something in a fashion magazine – the eighteenth-century stables, beautiful leather harness hanging up, hay protruding from an eighteenth century ironwork hayrick. Her ladyship Dodie was wearing a three-quarter length Afghan coat which emphasized her incredibly long legs. In the half light, her eyes completely dominated her face, like a young deer. I looked at Duncan but he seemed hardly to have seen her. His view was not helped by an extraordinary tartan pull-on hat, far too big for him, which he told me later was called a tamoshanter and which he wore as a mark of allegiance to a Scottish pop group called the Bay City Rollers, who he assured me were about to take the world by storm.

His eyes were entirely on the horse which, I must admit, looked decidedly under the weather. He could hardly stand, and while Duncan took his temperature I looked at his eyes. I tried to open his mouth, but it was stiff. I ran my hand over his flank. Everything was tense. Even his expression looked tense and worried, with his ears pricked forward.

'The tail, David. Have you noticed that it's not hanging straight?' Duncan volunteered, though it was less a question than a statement. At that moment, Seamus seemed to collapse. 'Know what I think, David? I think it looks like a classic case of tetanus! All we need now is to find a cut. We had a super lecture on tetanus last year. Covered all the animals that get it, sheep, cattle, pigs, even dogs. Did you know dogs even get it? Anyway, I remember this thing about a horse's tail. Although,' at this point he directed his tirade at Dodie, 'I can't believe you didn't get a horse like this vaccinated. You didn't, did you?'

I couldn't believe he had said anything quite so crass. But although his bedside manner might have been singularly lacking, his diagnosis was spot on. While he had been giving me the benefit of his expertise, I had been inspecting Seamus's hoofs for any sign of damage, having come to the same conclusion. No point in writing the colt's death certificate before being sure – because that's what a tetanus diagnosis probably was. But then I found it, a small infected wound on his foot, probably caused by nothing more dangerous than one of the sharp flints with which this part of the Weald was covered.

'Er . . . vaccination Lady Armistead?' I ventured. 'I don't suppose you remember if . . . when . . . ?'

'Well, d'you know, to be quite frank, I hadn't got around to it. Bit of a mistake I suppose,' she looked from one to the other of us, smiling.

'A verry expensive mistake your ladyship,' Duncan interrupted, his Scottish 'r's rolling menacingly. 'If my diagnosis is correct this horse will probably die and by the looks of him, he'll probably cost an arm and a leg.'

For a moment there was a terrible silence and I thought she was going to scream. I glared at Duncan but he just smiled back, delighted at having made an accurate diagnosis.

'Die? You don't mean that.' She turned from Duncan to me with her eyes suspiciously full of tears. 'Mr Grant? Surely now you're here you can give him something. He can't die. That's just not possible.'

I could hear the panic mounting in her voice.

'Well . . .' I hesitated. In these circumstances you don't want to raise hopes but at the same time, it's important not to be over pessimistic. After all I didn't want her to pass out, which looking at the colour of her face seemed a distinct possibility. 'Tetanus is very serious indeed. But he was standing when we arrived and that looks like fresh urine in his stall. So we may have got him in time.'

Tetanus, also known as lockjaw, is a disease caused by a germ which is commonly present in the faeces of animals – especially horses – and in the soil contaminated by those faeces. The spores can remain infectious for some years. Although completely harmless if it's eaten, if the bacterium gains entry through a wound it multiplies and produces a powerful toxin which causes nerve-system damage and a high mortality rate – around 90 per cent plus. It is easily prevented by a simple vaccine given when the horse is a foal and boosted a year later. Very often, as in this case, the germ gains entry through a wound in the hoof, and this may be difficult to find. We were lucky.

And what I had said was true. From infection to death is usually about five days, by which time the horse can no longer chew, as the jaw is too stiff. What Dodie had described as 'a turn' was a fit. These get progressively more distressing to the animal. As the disease gets worse the horse simply can't walk or even urinate because it can't adopt the posture to do so. Any noise may startle it and cause a tetanic convulsion, which is like a fit except that the limbs and the face become rigid. During these convulsions it easily falls on to its side and once down it is very difficult to get up again. Often they occur without even the stimulus of noise, and this is usually the beginning of the end.

The first thing to do was to open up the wound and drain it. This was something I was not prepared to let Duncan tackle. I pared away part of the hard skin, which is like thick nail, and found a small abscess underneath which I cleaned with antiseptic. Seamus was beyond even jerking his foot away. In the meantime Duncan was preparing a syringe of penicillin. Killing the germ stops the production of the toxin that is causing the symptoms. Next a further two injections; firstly a high dose of tetanus antitoxin injected into the jugular, then a sedative. In the meantime Duncan was setting up a saline drip which he suspended from a hayrack on the wall.

While all this was going on no one spoke. To give him his due, Duncan was pulling his weight, preparing and handing me things efficiently and calmly. Lady Armistead just paced up and down holding her head in her hands and saying nothing except 'I can't bear it, I just can't bear it,' repeatedly over and over again under her breath.

'Is there anyone who can stay with him tonight?' I asked when I had finished.

'I will. What do I have to do?'

'Try to keep him warm. Blankets, anything you've got. Get him to drink if you can. The drip should help, but he needs as much fluid as possible. I've given him a fairly hefty sedative that should last until the morning, by which time I'll be back to check on his progress. But tomorrow you should think about bringing in somebody to help you. He shouldn't be left alone.'

By now Duncan had packed everything away and filled a bucket from the tap outside in order to disinfect our boots when we got back to the car.

'I suppose my husband will have to be told.' The beautiful face turned itself towards me, as fearful as a child's.

'Yes,' I said, wondering if marriage to a much older man, however rich, was turning out to be something very different from what she had expected. 'I'm afraid this is going to be a long haul. And I should warn you, the chances are still very slim. Oh, and it might be as well to check up on your own tetanus records. It only takes a graze or a cut, particularly when you're mucking out.' As I said it, I realized they probably had staff to do that. 'Or even gardening.'

As we drove the mile up the drive to the main road, Duncan was for once silent. There would be a hard frost tonight, if not snow, I reckoned. Thank goodness I wasn't on duty. A full moon hovered above the hill to the east. It didn't look natural at all. Too big. Too yellow. When we reached the main road he turned to me, a triumphant expression on his face.

'That woman at the big house, Lady what-ever-her-name-was.'

'Armistead.'

'Aye. Well, I thought her face looked familiar and I've been racking my brains and I've just realized where I've seen her before. . . .'

'Have you, Duncan?'

'Aye. She's the spitting image of a girl my brother Alastair went out with last year. An air hostess with BOAC, she was and a real good looking lassie. Thought it was her at first. Jessie her name was, Alastair's girrlfriend I mean. I kept giving this one looks – perhaps you noticed – but she didn't react. So it can't have been her. And besides, the voice wasna right. Come to think of it you don't find many air hostesses among the aristocracy, do you? In fact I dinna ken I've heard of one. Have you David?'

'No, Duncan, I don't think I have.'

That evening I had had enough of company and decided to eat at a restaurant in town where the food wasn't fancy but which Keith had told me did just good solid English fare. And what I felt like was steak.

I ordered a 12-ounce sirloin and chips with a half a bottle of Spanish wine to wash it down, with Black Forest gateau to follow.

'Enjoy your meal, sir?' the waitress enquired, as I asked for the bill.

'Very much, thank you.'

She had her pad with her, and scribbled out the total there and then. I smiled and reached in my jacket for my wallet.

Oh no. I patted again. I couldn't believe it. The nightmare you've always dreaded. No wallet. Then I remembered. It was in my sports jacket which was hanging over a chair in the flat. I'd grabbed a thick coat because I hadn't want to drive.

There was nothing for it. I gave her a wave.

'Anything wrong, sir?' she said, looking worried.

'Well, er, yes. I've done something really stupid and forgotten my wallet. I could run back and get it, leave something with you . . .' But as I said it I realized I had nothing with me to leave.

'I'll just go and get the manager.'

As I watched her walk towards the service hatch, all those jokes about doing the washing-up flooded into my mind.

A portly man in his late forties made his way to my table.

'Louise tells me you've left your wallet at home.'

'That's right, but I'm very happy to—.'

He interrupted. 'That's no problem, sir. Just drop it in when you're next passing.'

I couldn't believe it. This man had never seen me before. I thanked him profusely and left. Sure enough the jacket was where I had left it. I didn't want to have this business hanging over me, so I went back straight away. I don't know whether it was the pleasure of having a good meal inside me, or the pleasure of knowing that there were still decent folk out there, but that night I slept like a log.

Chapter Six

About a week later I was surprised to see Miss Heskins' old Morris Traveller in the car park. I left Duncan with Peter, the other small-animal vet, and went to find Nick. We hadn't heard a peep from her since she had wanted us to give an autopsy to a fur ball a month or so back.

'So, Dr Lightfoot,' I said. 'I see young Horace is back to torment you again. A serious case of ear wax perhaps? Or do his claws need cutting?'

He laughed. 'A cut on his front leg. Nothing that a syringe full of penicillin won't cure.'

Suddenly I didn't feel like joking. 'Don't be so sure about cuts on legs, Nick. Pauline has just told me that the young horse I saw last week has died. Tetanus. Cut on the foot.'

We had done everything right, everything we could. But in the end, it wasn't enough. The line between life and death is very fine. Vaccinations are so commonplace now that it's easy to forget just how important they are, taking them for granted perhaps because they're free on the NHS. But animal vaccinations have to be paid for, whether it's a pig or a cat. And when an animal is young and healthy it's easy to forget that they are particularly vulnerable without the antibodies that both animals and humans build up with time.

In the case of Seamus, Lady Armistead's young horse, it was not even the money, just lack of thought. It wasn't a mistake she was likely to make again, that's for sure. Any animal, pet or farm, needs looking after with as much care as you would give a child.

That Christmas, with another assistant to take the strain and a student seeing practice, I had the whole week off. Christmas Day itself I spent with my parents – Rochester, where they still lived, was only forty-five minutes' drive from Canterbury and I always enjoyed spending time there – I am always surprised that the city isn't better known.

My parents had moved shortly after I left for the Royal Veterinary College in London. But the new house was only 100 yards from where we had lived when I was a boy. Then home had been a two up, two down terraced house built of brick. The new one was a 1930s semidetached villa with pink-painted pebbledash, which backed onto allotments that in turn backed onto a wild area leading up towards the old fort.

The hill beneath the fort was a mass of tunnels and strictly out of bounds when I was a boy. I was forbidden to go near them, let alone down them. Of course I did, often with Miffy, a neighbour's Jack Russell terrier, always reassuring myself with the old adage that had dominated life at school, 'Rules were made to be broken.'

Once I had the shock of my life when Miffy slipped off her lead and disappeared into the labyrinth. I could hear her barking, but the sound echoed around the tunnels so much that I couldn't tell where it was coming from. Then suddenly the barking stopped and I just knew she was dead. I started crying – just sat down on my haunches against the tunnel wall and cried like a baby. I was thirteen. The next thing I knew I felt a furry tongue licking the tears off my face. I don't know what had made her bark, or why she had suddenly decided to come back, though I suppose the sound of my crying made her inquisitive. She was used to hearing her name being called, but not the sound of crying.

Miffy was the reason I thought of becoming a vet. When she died a year or so later I was distraught and decided that, when I grew up, I wouldn't let dogs die. In fact there was nothing anyone could have done; it was just old age.

Rochester was a wonderful place to grow up. The streets backing onto the hill were all no-through roads so, unlike the hill itself, they were very safe to play in, with no cars, and everyone knew each other. Both my parents worked, which is why we didn't have a dog of our own, but there was always somewhere to go: Mrs Briggs at No. 53 or Mrs Harris in No. 39. It was all very Dickensian, little houses no more than 10 or 11 feet wide packed tightly together.

We children made our own entertainment, which changed as the years went by, from playing hopscotch and 'jacks' on the pavement – although this was really considered a girls' game – to football. We made 'dens' on the hill, where we collected wood for fires and cooked potatoes and sausages in the embers. The potatoes never cooked properly and the sausages were always burnt on the outside and raw in the middle, but smothered in tomato ketchup they tasted wonderful.

When we were older gangs of us would meet up and go on long cycle rides, usually west along the coast beyond the power station to beaches we thought nobody else knew about where there would be more fires and barbecues. Once we went across the estuary on the ferry to Southend – we must have cycled 70 miles that day.

It was a very close community. Throughout my childhood, except when I was walking Miffy, I was never alone. None of us were. There was always someone knocking at the door with the familiar 'Can David come and play Mrs Grant?' And I'd put on my shoes – in those days we never wore outdoor shoes inside the house – put on an old jumper or, if it was colder, my belted gabardine coat and I'd be off, disappearing in the morning and reappearing in time for tea, being 'up to no good' as my mother called it when she anxiously waved me goodbye.

No one thought of watching television, although I knew one family who had one. The first thing I remember seeing was the Coronation of the Queen in 1953 when we sat in rows, crammed into this family's front room. It was as exciting then as watching the moon landing later.

But by the late sixties everyone had television and my parents would watch it for hours. And Christmas 1969 was no exception. By then my mother had stopped working full-time and had acquired a dog, a black Labrador called Judy, who was the only excuse I could find to get away from sitting around the gas fire and watching the box. Because it was Christmas Day the streets were empty except for children pedalling spanking new bicycles, and Judy and I walked down through the town, past the vets in the High Street, where I had first convinced them to let me help out at weekends, past my old school, Sir Joseph Williamson's Mathematical School, founded in 1701 to give seamen's children an education, past the grocers where for years I had a Saturday job delivering groceries on a special bike with a basket on the front.

Boxing Day night at the Nightingales' was a fixture not to be missed. After Angie had left in the summer, the atmosphere in the house had begun to return to normal. I knew that it was nothing personal, simply that I had put Mrs Nightingale in a very difficult position. Now I was like the prodigal son and all was forgiven. She made a point of inviting me as Phil, her pilot son, and his new wife were coming. I had promised I would be there as Keith, her only other long-term lodger, and his fiancée Jenny were in Liverpool visiting her family. As I drove back from Rochester I wondered how the cockney lad was surviving a scouse Christmas.

In the Nightingale household there always seemed to be something to celebrate. This time it was Phil's prospective fatherhood. Of course I raised my glass of champagne like everybody else and slapped Phil on the back, but that night I lay in bed thinking about it: getting married was one thing, but the idea of someone of my generation being a father, that was something altogether different. I just couldn't imagine it.

My inability even to think of setting up home with one person had cut short at least two relationships, with Sally and Angie. And although I was fond of Caroline, I didn't really see that progressing any further either. The next academic year she was going to Toulouse as part of her degree. So that would be that I supposed. But this week at least, with Caroline back from college and me with a whole week off, we had until the New Year together.

Fortunately Mrs Nightingale had old-fashioned central heating that really worked, and my flat was always warm and welcoming. It was also beginning to feel more like home, with Janet's picture above the settee.

The five days left of the holiday passed in a haze of laziness. And as the days went on I became more and more comfortable with the idea that Caroline and I would do things together, get up, have breakfast, decide what to do, or what not to do. Even shopping for food, I discovered, was more fun with two. I began to understand how Keith and Jenny were happy just with each other's company. When I first arrived in Canterbury we had both been single, but since he'd fallen in love with Jenny I'd seen much less of him.

When the weather was fine, we did the mad things young people always do when they think they're in love. One afternoon we went to Herne Bay and spent hours walking along the beach, throwing pebbles into the sea, with no one to see us except seagulls and the occasional dog-walker. Then we huddled up in one of the shelters along the promenade, but only moving kept us warm in that wind. No one talked about the wind-chill factor in those days, but that didn't mean it didn't exist. When you're cold to the core, the only answer, we decided, was fish and chips, where even the neon sign looked warm. Cod and chips and steaming mugs of tea were followed by feeding a few shillings into fruit machines in an amusement arcade run by an old man who told us we were the only customers they'd had all day.

Another afternoon we went to Whitstable. It was like a page out of a history book. In the streets by the harbour, where they bring in the oyster dredgers, it still looked as it must have looked in Dickens' day. We egged each other on to eat oysters, and in the end we both tried one. At least this time I knew what I was eating, but I am sorry to say, I just couldn't take the idea of something live slipping down my throat. Perhaps it's the vet in me but I've never understood the appeal.

We didn't get to the place where Janet had painted the picture, the branch of the Stour. I thought it would probably be better once spring had arrived. I knew only too well from everyday practical experience that rain had made every-where too muddy for pleasure.

When we weren't out, Caroline worked on her dis-sertation, and I worked on learning Spanish. I had had a holiday with Keith and Jenny in Spain the year before and ever since, I had been determined to get to grips with it, enough to be able to have a proper conversation. The local tech was advertising evening classes, starting in January and among the basket-weaving, pottery and Scottish dancing, Caroline had spotted Spanish for beginners. In the meantime I had sent off for the *Daily Express Beginner's Spanish* Teach-It-Yourself book, designed for visitors to the newly popular tourist destination.

The time passed all too quickly. Keith and Jenny made sure they were back for New Year's Eve and, because I was on call, we had all agreed to join Theo's festivities at the Spotted Cow, preceded by supper at Selina and Nick's. It meant everyone else could walk home, without any need to cut down on the booze – all except me, of course – and Duncan, who had made it clear that an English New Year came a very poor second to a Scottish Hogmanay. I told him that there was no need for him to come with me but he was determined to 'play his part'.

When I dropped in at the hospital to ask Nick if there was anything I could bring, he immediately started talking to me about Horace. Apparently while I had been away the old ginger cat had become very ill indeed. 'And what's worse, I haven't a clue what's wrong with him or what to do,' he said. I had never seen Nick so worried by anything: the phrase laid-back might have been invented for him.

Within a couple of days the innocuous-looking wound on Horace's front leg had erupted all over with sores. Each sore had bunched-up hairs which you could pick off. He was literally covered in them. Nick had tried some steroids to see if that would help, this seemed to have the effect of making him even worse – he had developed all the signs of pneumonia. He was now fighting for his life in the hospital.

David Grant

It wasn't just Nick who was stuck for ideas; no one had ever seen anything like it. Horace was on a permanent drip with potent antibiotics. Frank had been quick to see the link between the steroids and the pneumonia, which was very astute since steroids were very widely used at that time and most skin conditions were given them. Nick told me that Frank thought it could well be a viral condition. A viral condition certainly fitted in with the steroids making it worse. All three small-animal experts were now involved.

New Year's Eve turned out to be fun but quiet – or so it seemed to me, maybe because I wasn't drinking. Selina had pushed the boat out on the food front, and the courses just kept coming and coming. Only when Keith looked at his watch and saw that it was half past eleven did we realize that we had to get going if we wanted to see the New Year in at the Spotted Cow. The night was clear and it was only a ten-minute walk, but even so, the rest of them only just made it. I drove, because I was still on call. At midnight the lid of the old piano in the corner was lifted and a bloke with a pork-pie hat began to play all the old songs, with everyone joining in. The evening ended with the song that was produced by Paul McCartney for Mary Hopkin, 'Those Were the Days My Friend'. And, yes, we thought they'd never end, but they had. The sixties were over. Long live the seventies. This is just how New Year's Eve should be, I remember thinking as Caroline and I made our way back to my flat.

Thirty years ago there was no New Year's Day bank holiday so the hospital was open for business. Although we hadn't gone to sleep until about three in the morning, I was as bright as a button, unlike everyone else I saw – excluding Miss Heskins, of course, whom I bumped into just before setting off on my rounds. Nick told me that, although she

80

lived in a village a good 10 miles away, she had been in twice a day since Horace was admitted to tempt him with what she called 'tasty morsels': bits of herring, kidney, chicken liver. You could see him trying to please her, but it looked like a lost cause. Pauline and Nick had both hinted, as diplomatically as possible, that she should prepare herself for the worst. Because he was on a drip, it had been decided that she should not take him out of his cage. Often over the next few days I would go into the ward where Horace was and see Miss Heskins' hunched figure poking bits of this and that through the bars and talking to him and scratching behind his ears.

Cats can live to a ripe old age, much older than dogs. I remember one which lived to be twenty-eight. Although he never had anything wrong with him, since the age of eighteen his owners had never been away on holiday, always thinking that if they did he was sure to die. Horace was only fourteen, and although he was a bit overweight through living a life of idleness and luxury with Miss Heskins, he should have had a good few years left.

One morning I went in and sat down beside her. She looked up at me and smiled. 'Do you think I'm a silly old woman, Mr Grant?'

'What makes you say that?'

'Because I don't know if I am doing the right thing. Keeping Horace alive.'

'Not if it's what you want Miss Heskins.'

'Now tell me the truth Mr Grant. Is Horace in pain? Dr Lightfoot says he isn't.'

'I'm pretty sure he's not in pain, Miss Heskins. I think he probably feels like we do if we've got the flu. Just very sleepy. It's not as if the sores seem to be troubling him. He'd be scratching them if they were and he's not.'

'I wouldn't want to prolong things for him unnecessarily.'

'Of course you wouldn't.'

'But it seems to me that he is trying. I'm sure I heard him give a little purr earlier on. And if he's trying, then it would be wrong to give up now, wouldn't it?'

I did my best to reassure her. But it wasn't as if I knew any more than the others did. Over the years I have often been faced with these situations and the only thing to do is to take your cue from the animal's owner. It was true that he wasn't in pain; if he had been, then my advice would have been different.

For a week Horace hovered between life and death. Then suddenly without warning or reason he began to perk up and eat, and not just Miss Heskins' tasty morsels. After two weeks he was well enough to go home. I happened to be in the hospital when his owner came to collect him. 'Well, Mr Grant. It was worth hanging on, wasn't it?' Her beaming face said it all.

'It certainly was, Miss Heskins,' I said. 'It certainly was.'

Just then Nick emerged, holding Horace in his wicker basket. The ginger cat had his face pressed up to the wire netting at the end and he presented an ear for stroking while Pauline prepared the bill. I could see she felt embarrassed handing it over. Two weeks in hospital, with all the associated drugs that Horace had had – including the steroids that hadn't done him any good – came to a lot, I knew.

Miss Heskins looked it over then looked up. 'That's very reasonable!'

We all smiled.

'Now Miss Heskins, if you are in the least bit worried about Horace, you must feel free to call. Any time, day or night.' It was Nick who said it, but it could have been me. He looked at me, and we smiled broad smiles.

She did call once, when Horace went off his food for a day or so. But that passed and was probably something entirely unconnected. We never did get to the bottom of the problem. All the tests proved inconclusive.

Then about ten years later, some time after I had begun specializing in skin conditions, I was sitting in a lecture hall at a congress in London and I saw the same condition described for the first time. The symptoms had been exactly the same.

It turned out that Frank's theory was right. What we had been looking at was a cat infected with cowpox virus, which in spite of its name is usually acquired by cats which are bitten by small rodents that they have been hunting. Horace was certainly a good mouser, as Miss Heskins had never failed to remind us. He was perfectly capable of taking on anything. Pity even the pigeon that fell foul of Horace on the war path. Most cases of cat pox get better just with nursing, we were told – unless, that is, they are given steroids, in which case pneumonia often develops and then it's touch and go. ·

Even though thousands of animals have passed through my hands over the years, there are some you never forget. Sometimes it's the animal itself, sometimes it's the owner. Sometimes, as with Horace and Miss Heskins, it's both. As I listened to the speaker describing cat pox, my mind immediately went back to Horace ten years earlier and a light went on. There was nothing for it, I had to phone Nick.

By now Nick Lightfoot was a senior academic at a prestigious university. But I was too late to surprise him. He already knew, he told me when I finally got through. He had seen the literature three months earlier. It wasn't just me who had remembered Horace it seemed.

I had always been interested in skin conditions, ever since I had disastrously misdiagnosed a puppy soon after I joined the practice, when Frank had fortunately put me right. For all his apparently easygoing nature, Frank was an extremely clever and well-read veterinary doctor. Nick had been right when he said that an apprenticeship with Frank and Alan was the best anyone could get.

Skin conditions are not limited to domestic animals, and about a month into the new year I came across an outbreak of orf – a viral skin disease that affects sheep – not that I knew it was that at the time. It happened on an isolated farm on the North Downs. It was around 9.00 p.m. and I had been nursing a pint of shandy in the Spotted Cow for what seemed for hours. Caroline had gone back to London, there was nothing interesting on television, and the regulars were not a bad lot and I felt like company.

'For you David.' The voice raised above the noisy hubbub of the bar was Theo's, with the phone in his hand. My heart sank. But when Alan's wife told me it was Dibber Martin with a difficult lambing I cheered up.

Dibber was an old shepherd. He couldn't have been much short of seventy and looked it. Bald as a coot, what he lacked on his head he made up for in the forest of whiskers that sprouted from his ears and nose.

A sense of humour is not something that I had noticed among farm hands before I got to know Dibber, but that was probably because I rarely saw them when they weren't working. As a vet, with 'all that larnin'', I was somebody farm hands doffed their caps to and that was it. I'd first come across him soon after I arrived in Canterbury – I can't remember the circumstances – probably a difficult lambing

just like this one. Then, when I was in Spain on holiday with
Keith and Jenny the previous year, I had noticed a familiar
face – or rather a familiar head. At first I couldn't place him.
He was dressed in creased white shorts, the kind that fifties
footballers used to wear, and a bright orange shirt covered
in palm trees. Then I had it. It was Dibber Martin, sitting at
a bar with a woman who, from the floral print dress and
sensible shoes I took to be Mrs Martin. But what were they
doing here?

Going abroad was not the common thing it is now. It
was the first time I had been abroad, if you didn't count a
German exchange at school. It was definitely Keith's first
time. Could it really be Dibber I wondered? There was
nothing for it but to go over.

''Af'r'noon, Misser Gran','' he said, his pale blue eyes
twinkling. His bald head was the colour of mahogany and
as shiny as a conker just prised from its shell. 'I knew t'was
you but didn't want to interrupt see, bein' as you'm wi' your
young friends.'

My offer of a drink was quickly accepted, however.
Dibber had clearly taken to the native wine with gusto – and
so he might at less than a shilling a bottle. I sat down while
the waiter busied around, clearing empty glasses.

His companion, who was introduced as Muriel, was not
his wife, it transpired later. That lady, it seemed, had died five
or so years previously and had been substantially older than
Dibber. On her death he had found himself the owner of a
small cottage and a surprisingly large building society
account. His current 'lady friend' lived in Sandgate and
several times a year, the two of them would go on coach trips
to the 'cong-ti-nang'. He was one of the first pensioners to
discover that you could live in Spain as cheaply as you could
at home. Now he only worked 'when it suited,' he said.

85

David Grant

When some time later I asked when he was going to make an honest woman of Muriel, he tapped his nose. 'If it ain't broke, don't mend it,' was his jaunty answer. As for his travels, what was the point, he said, of having money and not spending it? Unfortunately I was not in a position to know.

When Dibber had discovered the ewe in difficulties that night, he had brought her down from the hills in the back of an old Land Rover. He had tried to pull her lamb out himself, but when he put his arm in and found two he decided that was something not to attempt on his own. Two live lambs and a live ewe were worth calling the vet out for.

'Good to see you, Dibber,' I said as I pulled on my waders. It was a cold night.

'Well lad, I just hopes you can do yer stuff. She'm been a long time at it I reckon. Dry as a barley husk.'

Dibber looked very strange in the miserable conditions of an English winter in a lambing shed lit by one naked bulb. He and Muriel had just come back from a month on the Costa del Sol, he told me, as I managed to rotate the first lamb's head with the help of some hot water and soap flakes. Dibber had tried to do the same and he was stripped down to his vest. The lower half of his arm was the usual Dibber shade of mahogany to match his head, and the upper part was several shades paler than the sheep. He was making himself a roll up when I noticed what looked like blisters on his fingers.

'That's looks nasty, Dibber. Too much sun. You should be careful.'

'Nowt to do with sun, lad,' he replied. 'Only came up yesterday and I've been back three week come Sunday.'

With the lambs both safely delivered I gave the mother a quick check-up. She seemed none the worse for wear and was up and licking them both within minutes. In the corner of the lambing pen I noticed another ewe and a lamb about a week old.

'Why are they here, Dibber? The lamb looks a good size. Any problems?'

'Didn't seem to be sucking proper-like,' he explained. 'Feared the mother weren't givin' enough milk. Thought I'd best keep an eye on 'em.'

The pair were in a far corner of the barn where the thin light of the single light bulb didn't reach. I went to fetch my torch then climbed over the hay bales to take a proper look. The lamb was lying some way off from the mother who was on her side. It didn't take long to see what the problem was. Her teat was covered with crusty sores. I winced just looking at them. They must have been painful. No wonder she wasn't keen to suckle. And her udder looked suspiciously full and tender. Dibber was right, the lamb hadn't been having enough. I moved across to the lamb and saw that its mouth was covered in sores. As I held the trusting little fellow's head in my hands, something came back from the recesses of my mind. Orf, I said to myself under my breath. I think what we've got here is orf.

I called Dibber over and showed him. 'How many other ewes have you noticed like this?' I asked.

He scratched his bald head, then shook it. 'First I've seen,' he replied.

'Well, I don't like the look of her.'

I looked at my watch. It was 10.30. Was it too late to ring Alan? On balance I decided it was. He wasn't on call and the ewe didn't seem in any distress. I decided to get Alan's advice in the morning. In the meantime it was important that the lamb got enough to eat.

'Got any bottles Dibber?' I asked. This lamb would have to be hand-fed.

He had some being sterilized, he said, and he had enough milk.

For once I didn't have *Merck's Veterinary Manual* with me and it wasn't till I got back home that I was able to read up about it, but I was pretty sure I was right.

First thing in the morning I collared Alan, who was just on his way out to check up on some pigs that didn't seem to be putting on weight. As I gave him an account of what I had seen, Alan interrupted.

'Did you wash your hands David?'

I told him I had. Every vet learns how important it is to ensure that infection can't be transferred from one farm to another. And because my first experience as a qualified vet was with an outbreak of foot and mouth disease, where the dangers of cross contamination were devastating, I have never taken risks. Some of the older farmers used to laugh when I insisted on wearing a calving apron, for example, which reaches from below the knees to just under the chin, and I always wore gloves.

'Because the thing is,' Alan went on, 'orf is highly contagious, not only between the ewe and her offspring but to humans as well.'

It was then I remembered the sores on Dibber's fingers.

'Could well be,' said Alan. 'Anyway I think I'd better go up there right away. You go to the Hoskins' place and see to their pigs and I'll go and check up on these sheep.'

I caught up with him at lunchtime. The pigs would be fine, I told him, a touch of viral enteritis. As for the sheep, it was definitely orf, Alan had decided. Dibber hadn't been around, but he'd spoken to Doug, the regular shepherd, who confirmed that no other sheep had shown any signs of the crusty lesions. But as orf can stay in the ground for decades, Alan explained, it was crucial to vaccinate the whole flock.

'But we're talking about 500, Alan. The flock is one of the biggest in the practice.'

'I know. But it can't be helped. At least you'll have Duncan to help you.'

Doug had shown no signs of the disease himself, but Alan considered that his GP should be informed. There was no vaccination against orf for humans, it seemed. As for Dibber, like all viral diseases, it just had to run its course, though later he told me that the doctor recommended that he should be given antibiotics to prevent secondary infection, the same treatment as the sheep. In the meantime he should make sure not to touch his mouth and not to shake hands with anyone.

Alan had already ordered the vaccine from the manufacturers, he said. Although we had some in stock, we didn't have enough for 500 sheep. They had promised it would be there first thing next day.

The next morning definitely felt like spring. At least it had done in Mrs Nightingale's garden when I set off to pick up Duncan. Snowdrops poked their heads up underneath the pear tree beneath a pale blue sky. The sight that met our eyes when we arrived was like a scene from *The High Chaparral*, with sheep instead of cattle. I had never seen quite so many penned together. Doug, Dibber and their dogs had been working overtime. They had put together a run that led the sheep through like a conveyor belt. Duncan and I stood one each side. The sheep were let in one by one.

A vaccine is an attenuated – which means weakened – live virus. It had to be administered in a place which would not irritate the sheep and cause it to spread by licking. It occurs naturally, as I had seen, on the teat and the lips, both areas of great sensitivity and pain. Because the lamb's mouth is painful and because the mother won't let it suckle,

89

it not only jeopardizes the lamb's ability to feed, it also increases the risk of mastitis in the mother. Orf can be devastating if it gets a grip on a flock, with the lambs all having to be bottle fed because when the ewe isn't suckled, the milk will dry up.

The most out-of-the-way place on a sheep is the inner thigh. The special applicator first grazes the skin, then administers a drop of the vaccine. All quite simple – but first the sheep has to be turned over. It's easier if the sheep has horns, at least that gives you something to grab. Most of these didn't, which meant one of us had to grab the neck instead and using our own weight pull the sheep right over, so it was back on its haunches, leaning up against us. Then the other person would make the graze and drop in the vaccine. Pulling the sheep over and holding them still was backbreaking work and Duncan and I took it in turns. We could each manage about fifty at a go and then we'd change over. Duncan was in a surprisingly good mood; he said the place reminded him of home.

Before putting the sheep in the queue for vaccination, Doug had checked for any signs of disease, because any that were infected would have to be segregated and the lambs would have had to be bottle-fed, a nightmare in a flock that size. Luckily we had caught it very very early. But it was just pure luck that Dibber had happened to notice something was wrong, and had happened to mention it to me so that we were on to it in a flash, because with scabs on the mouth the virus can survive for years.

Usually with hard physical work, cold is not a problem, but it was that morning out on that windswept hillside. Even though the sun was shining we weren't really moving and inside the waders my feet got colder and colder, until I stopped feeling them. We had a thirty-minute break for tea and a sandwich at lunchtime, which Doug's wife brought up to the pens, and then it was back to the grindstone. The sun had already disappeared behind the hill when the last of the sheep came into the holding pen.

'What you need now is a whisky, lad. Nothing like it for warming the cockles,' Dibber informed me as I sluiced down my boots.

'Music to my ears, Dibber,' I replied.

'And what about your young friend?' he said, jerking his head towards Duncan.

'He doesn't drink,' I explained.

'Thought 'e were a strange fish,' Dibber snorted.

Half an hour later, however, Dibber, Duncan and I were sitting around the fire in his local pub, each with a glass of whisky. It turned out that Duncan's non-drinking stance was just that. He had wanted to create a good impression, he said. And telling me he didn't drink had made it easier not to succumb. But after his nostalgia for the Scottish moors had passed, 500 sheep on a windswept hill had done for his resolve. However, while Dibber and I had 'the other half' Duncan decided one was enough and asked for a hot drink. These days having a coffee in a pub is not so odd, but it was then. However, at a nod from Dibber Kathleen, the elderly landlady disappeared into her kitchen to see what she could do.

'Now there's a good 'un,' said Dibber.

'Aye, she is that,' agreed Duncan. 'Usually when I ask for a coffee I get a blank stare.'

'Bein' a furriner, he's not taken my meanin,' Dibber chuckles, giving me a hefty dig in the ribs. 'Eh lad?'

Then he made a sign that involved raising his right forearm at the elbow, which I recognized from Spain as referring to matters sexual, although it was an incongruous sight, as Dibber was wearing a large pair of sheepskin gloves which he refused to take off as he didn't believe in taking chances with the orf, he said. His bright eyes stared at me, his beetle eyebrows rising and falling like waves, willing me to understand.

'You don't mean . . . not you and Kathleen,' I gasped, suppressing a laugh.

'Shshsh,' he said, in a low growl, 'She'll hear.'

'But she canna be less than seventy,' Duncan whispered, having finally cottoned on.

'The best ones are over seventy, lad.'

'So you and your wife . . . ?' I hesitated. I had heard that Dibber's first wife had been twenty years older than him.

'S'right. She were the first. Never looked at a young 'un since. I were only fifty when we married, but truly her skin was as soft as a young girl's and not to put it in plain language, I could hardly keep up with her,' he added.

'Och, that's disgusting,' Duncan spluttered.

'Disgusting? What does a young ferret like you know about disgusting?'

It was time to leave, I decided. Fortunately Duncan had agreed to drive. I hustled him out of the pub so fast that I left my jacket behind. When I went back to get it, Kathleen had taken my place by the fire.

'Sorry about that, Dibber,' I said, grabbing the jacket.

'Don't you worry, lad,' he replied and gave me a wink as Kathleen bent down to push a log back onto the fire.

But I noticed that his gloves were still safely on his hands.

Chapter Seven

Duncan's inability to think before he spoke had already landed him in hot water. About a month after his arrival at the practice, there was a row. Although I wasn't there, Pauline was and duly relayed the scene to any interested parties, of which I was one.

Apparently Duncan didn't think that Frank had followed procedures for testing for antibiotic sensitivity before using antibiotics in a skin infection. 'What I'm saying Frank, and I trust you'll take this in the right spirit, is was it wise to skip the test? Our professors at college were adamant that it must be done. And I'm really surprised that you didna follow the literature in this one.'

Frank saw red, Pauline said. 'For a while he didn't say anything, just busied himself, collecting some papers together. Of course, I knew the signs. But Duncan didn't. And then when Duncan didn't stop, Frank came as near as I have ever heard him to shouting.'

'Young man,' he said. 'No doubt your professors had their reasons. But so have I. I believe you to be a very conscientious student and one who conducts meticulous research. I would suggest therefore you research my history. I think you will find that Frank Archer has the letters Dip. Bact. after his name. Do you know what that stands for? It stands for the Diploma in Bacteriology. I have had more experience of skin infections than you have had proverbial hot dinners, Duncan. And my empirical knowledge of this particular infection is that the antibiotic I intend using will have no ill effects whatsoever. Do I make myself clear?'

'Yes but Frank, it wouldna take that long to do the swab test and then if—'

'Enough. If you want to take this up with the other partners then you can put it on the agenda for the next meeting. Did you get that Pauline?' And with that he swept out.

I heard Duncan's version in the car a couple of weeks later when we were on our way to look at a budgerigar with a broken foot. Normally Frank was the avian specialist, but he had suddenly decided to take a week's break, skiing in the French Alps. He explained the last-minute nature of the holiday saying that he had the chance of a cheap deal. But word soon got around the practice that it was 'to get away from the student'.

Ever since he had arrived, Duncan had gone on about budgerigars. He knew more about them than most vets in the country, he said. Though that wasn't saying much, as what most vets knew about budgies in those days could be written on a postage stamp, and that included me. So when we got a call to see a budgerigar with a broken leg, Duncan was the obvious person to go. And I was down to go with him.

'You see, David, it's all a question of diet.'

'Is it?'

We were on our way to an address near the coast.

'Yes. The average budgerigar is fed the wrong kind of food. Over the year I have conducted a number of experiments. Did I tell ye that I breed budgerigars?'

'Yes, you did.'

'Well, when you breed them, several interesting things emerge between generations and because the incubation period is short, only eighteen days, it's possible to develop unusually close familial relationships.'

'Really.'

'Oh aye. Do you ken something, David, I enjoy talking to you. You're more approachable than some of the people in this practice. You listen and what's more you're interested. I suppose you heard what happened with Frank.'

'I did hear something.'

'Well, I put it to you. I'm here to learn good practice. And what do I learn? Short cuts. Frank actually put a dog on a course of antibiotics without giving it a swab test! And in my presence. And then he tried to justify his behaviour. Can you credit it? He broke the first cardinal rule of prescribing. What was the first lesson that we learned at college? Never trust to luck. And what's all this experience he's talking about but luck? You can't quantify experience, he says. No. And that's the trouble with it. Veterinary medicine is a science, David. And science can and should be tested. There is no place for luck in today's world.'

Over the last few weeks I had grown used to Duncan's monologues and had learned just to let them wash over me, but I was so irritated at this diatribe against the man who had taught me more than all my professors put together that I nearly didn't see a lorry pulling out of a side road. Luckily there was nothing coming and I managed to pull out around it. There was, I noted ruefully, a good deal to say for luck.

And Duncan was wrong about one thing. It was entirely normal and acceptable practice to give antibiotics for some skin conditions without swabbing and doing antibiotic sensitivity tests first. But his monologue had been so mind-numbing, and then with the lorry pulling out, I had no chance to put him right before he continued.

'Of course,' he went on, 'it's not just birds that I'm

David Grant

interested in. Oh no. Have you ever studied frogs, David? Fascinating creatures, frogs. Now I know that not many people have frogs as pets, but that may change. It's the life-cycle that is fascinating you see. Then there are gerbils. I have a particular fondness for gerbils and the symbiotic relationship they have with certain kinds of parasites. I find the word symbiotic very useful. Do you David? You should try using it more often. I find that when I use a word regularly it becomes part of my personality. Symbiotic is particularly useful when talking about parasites.'

When it came to parasites, I knew what it felt like. I supposed it came of spending your childhood surrounded by sheep. By the time we reached the outskirts of the village where the budgerigar lived, I had been drained of all energy.

'What I like about you David, is that you're willing to learn. Take today. You chose to come with me because you know you are weak on budgerigars and you wanted to expand your knowledge in the sure hands of someone with greater experience.'

Duncan was still talking as I rang the doorbell. I hadn't been convinced I had the right address. It was a prefab at the entrance to a small caravan park about half a mile from the coast. Home visits cost twice as much as coming to the surgery, but as the weather was too cold for birds to be taken out of doors, there wasn't much choice.

Of course Duncan was right about one thing. I did know nothing about budgerigars. I had had such a painful encounter with one shortly after I arrived in Canterbury, when I nearly killed a bird who attacked me just because I made a mess of cutting its claws, that I had spent the rest of my time trying to avoid them.

'Mr O'Donnell?'

'Who wants him?'

'I'm David Grant, the vet.'

'Why didn't you say so. Come in, won't you. The bird's through here.'

We followed the Irishman into the living room where Mrs O'Donnell was watching television.

'Will you turn that infernal thing off?' her husband shouted. 'Didn't you hear the doorbell, Mary. It's the vets come to see about Patsy. And I know they'll be wanting a cup of tea.'

'Did you say Patsy, Mr O'Donnell?' Duncan had decided to speak.

'I did young man.'

'But I understood from the records that your budgerigar was a male.'

'And so he is. So he is.'

'But Patsy . . . ?'

'Ho!' the old man laughed. 'And you were thinking it was a girl's name. No, no. Maybe in Scotland, but not in Ireland,' he said with a glint in his eye. 'He was named after my brother Patsy. Who was named after my father before him and his father before him.' Then added, 'But don't you be telling me the sex of a bird makes a bat's fart of difference to a broken leg.'

Mrs O'Donnell soon appeared with a pot of tea and slices of what looked like fruit cake. 'Irish brack,' she said proudly as I congratulated her on her baking. 'From a recipe I had from my mother, who had it from hers. It's made with tea, you know. No eggs. It's the tea that makes it light.'

While Mrs O'Donnell fussed around, getting sugar for Duncan and then a spoon, Mr O'Donnell was warming to his don't-take-me-for-a stupid-Irishman theme. 'Although I appreciate the care you obviously intend taking with Patsy

David Grant

here, I find it hard to see why a poor budgerigar that weighs less than a blackbird's egg needs the two of yous.'

I explained that my colleague had greater experience than I had with budgerigars. That I was more familiar with pigs and cows.

Patsy was an old budgie who had somehow got his right leg trapped in the bars of his cage and had a simple break of the main bone. He didn't seem too put out by the situation and was hopping about on his perch on one leg and squawking. This was one occasion when I intended to let Duncan do everything.

Pasty's owner was the epitome of the gentle giant. He told us that he had come over from Ireland before the war to work in the London docks. Then, when war was declared, he'd moved to the naval dockyard at Chatham. His children had been born in Kent, and now their first grandson had just been born. Although they went back to Ireland for holidays, England was their home now. They had always loved caravan holidays and when a house on a caravan park had come up for sale in their favourite part of Kent, it was decided. It was a bit draughty, Mr O'Donnell explained, but as it was halfway between a house and a caravan so what should you expect?

Meanwhile the bird hopped around his perch on one leg, giving us malevolent looks and intermittently squawking to let us know he knew we were there. The family history over, I decided to get on with the job. Patsy turned out to be very wriggly and it was hard to examine the leg.

'Och, give him to me,' Duncan said, failing to mask the exasperation in his voice. 'This is how you do it David,' and he cupped his hands and expertly trapped the bird inside upside down. Pulling the leg through a gap between his fingers the break was easy to see. 'I'll put a wee splint on it now that you know how to restrain the patient,' he said with the air of a hospital consultant doing the grand rounds.

Cupping my hands over my stomach I was able to trap Patsy after which Duncan gently pulled the leg through. Using two match sticks and some tape a 'wee' splint was fashioned in two minutes and Patsy hopped back into his cage looking like something out of a cartoon. Cue for another cup of tea.

On the way back to the hospital Duncan quizzed me as to how long budgie fractures take to heal.

'I thought you would have known that Duncan. You are, after all, the budgerigar expert.'

He nodded. 'Aye, well, I should say we'll have stability by the time I go back to college at the end the month.'

I decided not to say anything further. Duncan was clearly an irony-free zone. But if I imagined the silence would continue I was mistaken.

'I have to tell you, David, that I'm a wee bit surprised you're not up to scratch on budgies – Frostie's lectures were super. Did you not go to them?' Frostie was the nickname of the budgie expert at college. We had had all of three lectures on the budgie and I had missed all but one because they conflicted with my athletics training and I gave them a low priority.

Athletics had been rather on my mind recently as I had been contacted by the AAA – the Amateur Athletics Association – asking if I would run in a friendly at the beginning of the season. Although I had done no training since the previous summer, in the end I had said yes. It would be a chance to see some of my old athletics friends. The date was a long way ahead and I wasn't committing myself to anything long-term. It was just a one-off.

*

The phone went at 4.30. A calving down on the marshes. I hadn't slept well. All night the wind had been lashing at the windows. And now that I was truly awake I could hear that it was rain. I made a dash for the car and switched on the ignition, and the Anglia stuttered into life.

Calving is difficult at the best of times. The sheer physical energy expended in pulling a reluctant calf into the world is like nothing else. But at five in the morning in late February? I must be mad, I thought, as I took the ring road at well over the limit. This was an emergency, and anyway, no one in their right mind would be out on a night like this. Not even Ken Hitchens.

The northern tip of Kent was once an island, and what used to be the sea that separated it from the mainland is now reclaimed marshland criss-crossed with drainage dikes. Villages are few and far between, and those that are there are built on slight hills, little more than dry bumps. Because of the marsh, there was no new building – all the available land had long since been used up. Fortunately after nearly two years I knew my way around, though to anyone else Kent is a labyrinth of unsignposted roads. We used to joke that they took the signs down when Kent was under threat of German invasion and forgot to put them back after the war, but it may be true. There is nowhere else in England where the minor roads are totally unsignposted. And the same is as true today as it was thirty years ago.

I reached the farm at around six o'clock. If anything the sky had grown darker since I left home and by the time I reached the farm, it was sheeting down. Martin Fenwyck was waiting for me, sheltering in a shed by the road. He was a dour man, with a head that seemed too big for his body. He was carrying a hurricane lamp. 'The road up ahead is flooded so we can't get nearer than this. It's a good mile I'm

Still Practising

afraid. You better get what you need.'

I opened the boot of the Anglia and put on my waders. Then off came my jumper, shirt and vest. In those days I rarely felt the cold, but this was bad. The calving apron was made of rubber and I couldn't work out which was worse, the cold of the rubber or the cold of the rain. I jammed the torch into the hinge of the boot, found the calving ropes and put them in a duffel bag which I slung over my shoulder. I passed Martyn the bucket and without saying anything he filled it with water. He knew the drill. Then I retrieved the torch, tucked a packet of soap flakes under that arm and picked up the bucket of water with the other. Martyn carried another bucket.

Cow pasture is bad enough to walk on at the best of times, always churned up at the gates and wherever there is water. But in those fields down by the marsh, there is water everywhere. Every footstep is a booby trap. The holes in the mud can be 9 inches deep. What looks like firm ground can turn out to be like quicksand. Sometimes the mud itself can cling to your boot and refuse to let go. Walking a mile or more on land like this is exhausting and makes running the 200 metres seem like child's play.

It was a good forty-five minutes before we reached Hyacinth, as she was called. We walked in near silence, Martyn concentrating on leading the way and avoiding too many obstacles, me just thinking that enough was enough and that I must be mad to be doing this and I had to think seriously about changing my job.

By now the level of the water at the dike beside the cow had risen and to reach her we had to wade the final 20 yards through water that reached well above my knees. Martyn went in front of me. He knew where the land dipped and rose. Although I was soaked through to the skin already, the last thing either of us wanted at this stage was a vet who was unable to move because his waders were full of water.

It was over two hours since Martyn had left her and, as I had suspected, she was quite dry. I soaped my arm up and I put my hand in, and immediately felt a large head and two legs. So the calf was presenting properly, that wasn't the problem. The problem, I suspected was that it was large, just too large for Hyacinth to push out on her own. What was needed now was sheer brute strength. I felt for the first joint of each leg, and the next one up, to see if it was the front leg or the back. All was well. Head and two front legs. I gave a tug, but nothing happened. Nothing for it but to get the calving ropes on. I took off the duffel bag and got the ropes, attaching one on each leg above the hoof and then one around the head, behind the ears and into the mouth to ensure there was no pressure on the neck or windpipe. I put an extra handful of soapflakes in, then handed two ropes to Martyn, keeping the one on the head myself.

'Okay. Steady as she goes, one, two, three, pull.' I yelled.

Nothing.

'Okay, again. One, two, three, pull.'

After about five minutes I put my hand up again to check if there had been any movement. Hardly anything. Then, just as I was about to withdraw, I felt the beginnings of a contraction.

'Okay, Martyn,' I shouted as I hastily withdrew my arm. 'Now. One, two, three, pull.'

And with that everything began to move. Hyacinth gave a long, low moan and within two minutes her calf was safely on the ground and she was nuzzling it into life.

'A heifer. Your lucky day.'

After checking that all was well, I gathered up the ropes

and put them back in the duffel bag, all ready for the practice washing machine. The wind flapped at the bottom of my calving apron and I began to shiver. I realized that the rain had stopped.

The dawn was up, the birds had gone quiet, just as they do for the few minutes before the sun rises, and as we watched, the horizon was broken by fire. Suddenly life didn't seem so bad. Another live animal brought into the world and the prospect of breakfast and a hot bath to the accompaniment of Mahler's Fifth Symphony, which I had just added to my burgeoning record collection. I had heard it on the radio one morning driving down the Roman road towards the Romney Marsh. I didn't know what it was, and although it was not my usual kind of music I just knew it was good. I was driving to a farm out on the Weald and just praying I wouldn't get there before the music ended and they said who the composer was. So when I was within a half a mile of the farm, I pulled up at the side of the road and listened until it came to an end. Mahler's Fifth Symphony. For me, it doesn't matter whether a piece of music is classical, something by the Beatles or a torch song by one of the greats. Hearing them for the first time, there's a recognition that this is something great and it makes me want to jump up.

It was typical late February weather – one day warm enough to sit outside the pub, basking in the noonday sunshine, the next cold enough for Mrs Nightingale to turn the central heating up. The day before Duncan was due to leave, we were right on the border of the area covered by the practice, down in the south near Romney Marsh where I'd been doing a bit of TT testing. I decided to phone in to see if it was best to leave the rest of the herd until the weather improved.

Charles said he thought it safest to start making our way back. Then he said that Frank wanted a quick word.

'How is it down there?'

'Pretty bad, and getting worse I should say. Anything up?'

'Just that a friend of mine, my solicitor in fact, is in the next village to you and says he has a ewe with a prolapsed uterus. Usually of course I'd do it myself, but with this weather, and with you being there . . .'

'Of course, Frank. No problem.'

Edgar Peploe had a small flock of Jacob's sheep, an old breed usually kept for their wool which is a dark brown. He kept them in a field on one side of a small country house. They lived out all year round, with just a lean-to for shelter in bad weather.

All day Duncan had been mocking my 'sassenach' thick jacket and even thicker jumper, my mother's Christmas present. He was dressed in his usual sports jacket, tie and green cord trousers, topped with a standard issue brown cotton coat for use when examining animals. His only acknowledgement of the weather was his tamoshanter.

It was only about 8 miles from where we were, but my trusty Ford Anglia had been standing all day and although I turned the heater up to full, the temperature never rose beyond zero. Inside or outside the car, it was freezing.

'OK, Duncan, so what do you know about a prolapsed uterus?' I said, deciding to give him a taste of his own medicine.

The short answer was, not much. Luckily it was a subject I knew quite a lot about – at least in cows. It had come up in my final oral examination and I had made a complete hash of my answer. You never forget something like that.

'I do know that you canna take your time. I know that if you don't get it back in quickly they'll likely die.'

'Ever seen one?'

'No. But it must be easier than a cow.'

It will be for me, Duncan, I thought to myself. But not, I'm afraid, for you.

We found the ewe buried in straw under the lean-to, sheltered from the blizzard. The womb had expelled itself when she had given birth, and now hung between her legs like a deflated balloon. There was no point cleaning it yet. I quickly turned her upside down, put ropes around her back legs and gently lifted her up, tying the ropes behind Duncan's neck.

'Stand up Duncan, so I've got a bit of room to work.'

Of course he had been right about a sheep being easier, because you work on it the easy way up – the problem with a cow is that putting the womb back in is a fight against gravity, because you can't turn her over. You must also keep the womb clear of the ground. It's definitely not something you can do on your own. The first thing I had to do was to clean off the straw and anything else it had collected on its surface. Fortunately Duncan was quite tall, so with the ewe upside down at chest height it wasn't too difficult to gently massage the balloon back in, aided by liberal amounts of soap flakes and warm water that the solicitor had carried out from the house in a large white enamel jug, together with a kettle full of boiling water to top it up when it got cold.

Once the womb was back inside, I fashioned a truss of binder twine which I then wound round her legs, criss-crossing under and over her tail to keep it from falling out again. If I'd had a camera, this would have been a moment to capture – Duncan, with ropes around his neck taking the weight of a full-grown sheep, standing in his sports-jacket covered with a flimsy cotton overall against a backdrop that would have done justice to an Alpine postcard, his face a whiter shade of pale tinged with blue and his teeth chattering, all topped with a tamoshanter.

Edgar Peploe returned just as we had finished making our patient comfortable in the straw. 'Good timing,' he said, then turned to Duncan. 'I was going to suggest crumpets and tea, but looking at you, young man, a large whisky might be more in order.'

'Is this all they issue you with?' Mr Peploe asked, as he took Duncan's thin brown coat and hung it on a coat hanger over the Aga. We were in the kitchen as the drawing room, Mr Peploe had said, was 'bloody freezing'. He lived there on his own, with only a housekeeper for company.

'I'm from Scotland. I dinna feel the cold,' Duncan said, warming his hands on the Aga.

'Don't feel the cold! Don't be so bloody ridiculous. You're lucky not to have got hypothermia m'boy. You might have a degree in veterinary medicine, but you obviously haven't got one in common sense.'

Mr Peploe was quite at home in the kitchen and busied himself toasting crumpets and spreading them with so much butter that when we bit into them, it trickled down our chins. He poured Duncan a large tumbler of whisky which revived his spirits somewhat, particularly when he discovered that it was a 15-year-old malt. Reluctantly I turned down the offer and stuck to tea with plenty of sugar – the roads were sure to be lethal and I didn't want to take any risks with my concentration.

'Now,' Edgar said as we were about to leave, 'no doubt you will think me an old fuddy duddy, but I'd feel happier if you'd take these with you,' and he handed me an old blanket and a shovel. 'Just in case you know. The shovel is obvious and the blanket has two functions. The first one, also obvious, for warmth. Your friend could probably do with that. Less obviously you can use it if you have to dig yourselves out. Even when you can't move forward you can usually put her into reverse. Reverse onto the blanket and you've got some sort of purchase.'

While Duncan disinfected the waders I decided to check on the ewe. The snow was still falling and our footsteps from less than an hour earlier were already merely dents.

'Do you want the good news or the bad news?' I said when I got back to the car. Duncan was already sitting inside wrapped in the blanket. He wound down the window and looked up at me quizzically. 'The good news is that you are about to double your experience of this particular condition. The bad news is that we've got to do it all again.'

This time the fault had been mine. My hands had been too cold and I hadn't made the truss tight enough. The womb had simply fallen out again. While Duncan put on his waders again, I went back to the house for more water. Fortunately, second time around the womb went back in quickly. Edgar Peploe stood at the door to see us off, this time for good.

'Just give her a look every half hour,' I called. 'And if it come out again, I'll send out my colleague, now that he knows how to do it!'

When Edgar had offered us the shovel I didn't really think we'd have to use it. But we did. On the narrow lanes that cut deep into the hillsides on the way north, drifting snow could easily block the way. And several times Duncan had to get out and push us out of several snow drifts. Somehow he never suggested using the blanket for its alternative purpose; it remained dry and warm in the front seat.

It took us two hours to get back to the hospital. The sudden change in the weather had taken the roads authorities by surprise. The roads weren't gritted, bad enough on the side roads but even worse in the main road, because the traffic was down to one lane, a lorry having skidded across a junction.

My garrulous companion of recent weeks was no more. Duncan was a picture of miserable silence. The offer of a hot toddy at the Spotted Cow fell on deaf ears. He was off for a hot bath and an early night, he told me.

Next morning, the snow was still lying. It was school half-term, and the park across the road from where I lived was full of children enjoying the fun. But if I thought there would be no calls I was mistaken. There were plenty of home calls, it being too cold to bring animals to the hospital. And of course, there was a budgie.

'Nothing you can't handle,' Frank said. 'Especially with our budgie specialist with you. His last day isn't it?' I nodded. 'Hmmm. Well, Madeleine Ormerod is one of our favourite clients. Unfortunately I won't be able to deal with her myself as I'm speaking at a symposium in London.' There was something in his voice I couldn't quite decipher. I decided it was the relief that Duncan wouldn't be there when he got back.

Miss Ormerod was a retired actress, who Pauline reliably informed me had been a big star in the fifties, and her budgerigar Larry had apparently caught one of his claws on the bars of the cage and ripped it out.

Although it was only eleven in the morning, the woman who opened the door had, I judged, already had one too many. She was wearing a floor-length dress of a shiny material, which I realize now was a kimono, but then just assumed was some sort of dressing gown. Her face was liberally, though not accurately, powdered and the line of the lipstick didn't correspond to the line of her mouth. She was in a state of near hysteria.

'He's dying, I tell you. Dying,' she cried, and grabbing Duncan's arm propelled him into the living room.

'Pull yourself together woman, he's not,' said Duncan who was peering into a cage designed to resemble an oriental temple, where the budgie in question was perched on a wooden bar, spattered with blood. On the floor of the cage was a saucer.

'What's in here?' asked Duncan.

'Cognac, of course. For the pain, darling. I could hardly give him aspirin could I?' The bleeding had stopped and I was all for doing nothing but Duncan insisted on getting the bird out and cleaning it up. It perched on his finger happily enough, then seemed to wobble and lurch.

'There. What did I tell you,' his mistress shrieked. 'He's dying, dying. Dear Larry,' she said, by this time nearly in tears. 'He has strutted and fretted his hour upon the stage. But now no more,' and she went off to the kitchen exclaiming, 'Cognac, cognac, my kingdom for a cognac.'

Her exit seemed to act as a cue for her bird and he immediately perked up and hopped back on his perch. Duncan meanwhile calmly helped himself to the brandy.

'Ugh,' he said, wrinkling up his nose. 'Spanish.'

It was a good five minutes before Miss Ormerod returned. The red kimono had been replaced by one in black. In the meantime Duncan had cleaned up Larry's leg. He just needed a bit of time to readjust his balance, he said, and he'd be fine. Miss Ormerod confessed she would have liked to have offered us tea but she was sorry she had no milk. Perhaps we could like to join her in a glass of cognac? We declined.

David Grant

Duncan's time with us was at an end. I had completely forgotten about our other budgerigar but Duncan hadn't. Patsy's leg would have healed by now, he reckoned, and it was just a mile or two further on.

This time Mr O'Donnell greeted us with smiles. The kettle had just boiled, he said. He apologized for their being no brack, but Mrs O'Donnell was visiting their latest grandson. He could offer us Wagon Wheels and chocolate digestives instead.

With me doing the assistant's job, holding Patsy upside down in my cupped hands, Duncan carefully unravelled the splint he'd put on three weeks earlier to reveal that the leg had healed straight and strong.

'Okey-dokey, you can release him now David,' he said, beaming.

I opened my hands and Patsy flapped his wings, did a quick circle of the room before coming to land on top of the cage. But something was wrong. For a moment I couldn't work it out. Then it became clear. The leg was set the wrong way round.

I looked at Duncan. He had gone bright red and for once wasn't saying a thing.

'Well,' I said, addressing myself to Mr O'Donnell, 'the leg seems to have swivelled round – although he can perch quite well.' I paused, but no one said anything. 'But to get it just right,' I continued in a calm and matter-of-fact voice, 'I think it would be best to rebreak the leg and set it again.' But the gentle giant would have none of it. It would be an awful lot of trouble for both us and the bird, he said. And he went over to the cage and Patsy jumped onto his finger.

'Sure he can perch quite well and Mrs O'Donnell will never notice a thing – she's awful short-sighted!'

Still Practising

On the way back to base I waited for Duncan to say something. He said nothing.

'Odd about that leg,' I remarked eventually as we neared the practice. 'If I were you Duncan, and I hope you take this in the spirit it is intended, I would gen up on budgie biodynamics. You never know when it might come in useful. Perhaps Frostie forgot to point out the way a budgie's leg should go. Or perhaps you missed that particular lecture? You see the great thing to remember about budgie legs, Duncan, is that they share certain similarities with other birds' legs. That is to say, they bend backwards, Duncan. You know, the opposite of us humans.'

After I'd had my five minutes of fun I said, 'Look, I don't think there's any need to tell anyone about this.' After all the client was happy. And it was his last day. To say he was grateful is an understatement.

'What do you say to a farewell drink,' I suggested as we neared the practice. For once I had a free evening ahead of me. For all my irritation, I had grown to like 'the Scottish git' as Keith affectionately called him. He had his heart in the right place, and for keenness he couldn't be beaten.

'I really envy you your job,' he admitted as we downed our third pint of the evening. 'And I feel I've learned from you, David. Aye, that's for sure.'

'What on earth can you have learned from me?'

'Listening, David, listening. I've heard you listen to what the farmers have to say before doing anything else. We were never taught how important that is. It made me realize that I talk too much. And I should like to thank you for that. It's a lesson I shall never forget.'

Chapter Eight

I have always been fond of sheep, they are really lovely animals. They are not aggressive, they are a manageable size and, from the veterinary perspective they get some quite fascinating problems. And as for lambing, bringing a new life into the world never ceases to be a tremendous thrill. Sometimes that spring, when I was driving back from a job and not in a rush, I would stop the car beside a field of lambs and just watch them running about, shy yet curious, not straying too far from their mothers. No matter how low I felt, watching a field of lambs would always set me right.

Friends of mine who are doing large-animal veterinary practice now say there is hardly any sheep work because sheep are worth absolutely nothing, so they just don't get called out. Although I know that sheep farmers, like all farmers, are far more switched on than they used to be, I can't believe that self-help methods have changed very much and I suspect that the situation is far from satisfactory.

Sometimes a farmer has no option but to call a vet if his animals are to survive. Sheep bloat is one of these situations. The reasons for sheep bloat are similar to those in cows: too much rich pasture, particularly clover. Certain types of pasture are known to be risky, and the way to lessen the risk is not to let them eat too much, usually by a method called strip grazing, where they're given only a small part of a field or pasture at a time, the rest being fenced off. Unlike most emergencies, which in my experience always seem to happen at night, my first and only experience of sheep bloat was in broad daylight on a beautiful Sunday morning shortly after Easter. Although I had dealt with Major Boyce's bloated cow, this was very different, if only in terms of sheer numbers. A flock of about thirty or forty sheep had broken through a fence into a meadow that was rich in clover and had been stuffing themselves on the new grass.

Although the meadow lay near to the house, the farmer had been somewhere else on the farm and it was his wife who noticed something was wrong. The sheep didn't seem to be moving, so she walked up from the house to see what was happening. When she saw the sheep lying on their sides, their bellies all puffed up, she must have had a terrible shock. This was long before the days of mobile phones, and as she couldn't reach her husband she had called the practice immediately.

The field the sheep had broken into sloped down towards a stream and beyond that was the house, which lay at the edge of the village, no more really than a collection of houses around a church. The house itself was very old, a black and white Tudor manor house. None of the black timbers was quite parallel and the uprights were bisected here and there by horizontal beams, all of which gave the house the appearance of instability, though it had probably looked like that for more than 400 years. Part of the roof came right down to within about 6 feet of the ground and was green with moss. The garden at the front was planted with an intricate pattern of low box hedges. Looking from the field above, what really struck me that morning was the staggered line of the roofs of the house and various outbuildings behind it, all different heights and angles, with two round oast houses, their wind fins pointing in different

113

directions. It was really idyllic. When I first saw it I remember thinking, Wow, this could be used in a film.

By the time I got there the farmer had arrived and was busy rounding up the sheep that could still move with his dog, Floss.

Alan had gone through with me exactly what I had to do. Fortunately it was pretty much the same as for cow bloat: first, stick a large bore needle into the stomach to release as much gas as possible, then put a stomach tube down and pour in bloat drench. Major Boyce's cow had been too far gone for bloat drench, but most of these sheep were not in that state. It is essentially a special blend of vegetable oils that break up the gaseous froth that is filling the stomach. Each animal only needs a relatively small amount. Though I had never used it before, we always carried some with us in the boots of our cars.

It was a bizarre sight, about twelve sheep lying scattered over the meadow. Walking among them was an eerie experience because of the silence. They couldn't bleat or make any sound at all, as they could hardly breathe. This situation improved as soon as the gas was released. The procedure was simple. After the gas had escaped through the hole I made in their bellies with the needle, the farmer, Simon Battersby, held them down while I stuffed a tube down their throats and poured in the bloat drench through a funnel.

As soon as each one was done and they were back on their feet, Floss shepherded them into a holding pen to keep them under observation. In the meantime, a farm hand was busy repairing the fence where they had broken through.

What struck me was the haphazard nature of it all. Here was this beautiful village, basking in the first really warm sunshine of the year on a beautiful Sunday morning with the church bells ringing, and tragedy had struck – or could so easily have done. It was pure chance that Mrs Battersby had looked out of the window; and instinct rather than any knowledge that made her think something was wrong. A hour later, probably none of them would have survived and for a farmer to lose twenty to thirty sheep at a go would have been an absolute disaster.

The hedges told their own story as spring turned to early summer. Primroses gave way to cow parsley, bluebells to red campion and dog roses clambered up hedges that had grown bushy with new growth. I have never lost my love of the countryside and sometimes I think it would have been nice to be a partner in a country practice, but then I wouldn't have been able to follow my speciality. Life doesn't always work out the way you think it's going to.

My mind often strayed to Sister Theresa, the beautiful Irish nun I had met on my first visit to her convent, shortly after I first arrived in Canterbury. Surely, when she was a young girl living in the south-west of Ireland, skipping in the playground, climbing trees, or even perhaps kissing boys, she hadn't imagined she would become a nun. What had happened in her life to have brought her here? As it happened, a few days later I was called out to the convent. I hadn't been there for some time – which in a way shouldn't have surprised me. The sisters looked after their Jersey herd with as much care as if they had been children. Nor did they believe in spending money they didn't have to. Although I always looked out for Sister Theresa during my rare visits, I had always been disappointed, but I had never forgotten the faraway look she had given me the only time we had ever spoken. The other sisters seemed to lose their identify under the cowls of their brown habits, which is probably why they wore them. But Sister Theresa's beauty shone out. I couldn't understand why I had never seen her again. Had she left the convent?

It was a Saturday night in early summer, yet another weekend duty. It seemed most weekends were taken up with work one way or another, at least the ones that were hot and sunny, when everyone else seemed to be making for the beach. Another of Nick's hobbies turned out to be sailing. Naturally our weekends off rarely coincided but the one time they did there were gale warnings, hovercraft crossings were cancelled and even action-man Nick conceded that it was too dangerous to go out on the briny. But I must say I quite enjoyed the weekend, sitting in the beach hut they had rented for the summer just along from where Nick moored his sailing dinghy. Selina had even set up a Primus stove and, as usual, concocted marvellous things out of nothing, though she could never get me to eat the seafood she and her friends collected among the rocks on the shore; fish and chips was still hard to beat, I reckoned. That weekend they had invited yet another girl down, though I had begun to suspect that these 'dates' were more for the girls' benefit than mine. This one was a complete non-starter. Maddy had just split up from her boyfriend and was well named. She spent half her time in tears and the rest taking lone walks along the beach while we played poker and told raucous stories.

Nick was determined that I should experience the thrill of driving in Selina's soft-top MGB. His own car was a souped-up Mini which he kept for rallies. He drove as if his life depended on it, much faster than I did, yet he had never been stopped by Ken Hitchens or one of his cronies. But then again, as a small-animal vet he wasn't doing the 500 miles a week that I was.

If my weekends off were always heralded by thunderclaps as torrential rain set it, when I was on call it was different. The evening I set off for the convent was balmy, with the temperature still in the seventies. A steady stream of traffic was heading back into town as I drove in the opposite direction, east towards the coast. It was still hot enough for a heat shimmer to be seen on the roads and the air was very still. The convent lay on the outer edge of the practice area and village after village that I drove through on my way had groups of young people spilling out into the garden frontage with pints of frothy Kentish ale in their hands.

As usual, the gate of the convent was opened by Sister Maria Assumpta, who led me behind the chapel towards the farm.

'So, Mr Grant again, is it?' she said in her soft Irish voice.'

''Fraid so, sister. It's that home made wine you keep giving me.'

'Is it so.'

Conversation with Sister Maria Assumpta was always slow.

'What do you make it from?'

'Why grapes, Mr Grant. What did you think we made it from? We may be nuns but we're not stupid you know.'

'I didn't know you had a vineyard, sister.'

'It's not a vineyard, it's three indoor vines, planted during the First World War. There was no wine, you see, for Communion.'

'And do you still drink it, Sister?'

'God bless you, no. The convent wine has never been drunk by a member of the order.'

'But I thought you said . . .'

'I told you why we'd planted the vines. But it was a

good few years before they started producing grapes, and by then the war was over.'

We had reached the cowshed and I still hadn't plucked up courage to ask about Sister Theresa.

'Sister Claudia is in charge of the farm now,' she said, as another nun glided up beside us. 'So I will leave you in her capable hands.'

Sister Claudia was no Sister Theresa I noted. She was in her middle fifties, wore pale horn-rimmed glasses and seemed very cheerful and contented. She surely would know what had happened to her predecessor I thought, as I trudged across the deep straw bedding past curious cud-chewing Jersey cows in her wake.

'Have you worked with the cows long?' I ventured as a start to what I hoped would be an interesting conversation.

'Bless you, no.'

'The sister who was in charge of the cows before – now what was her name – er, Sister Theresa. What happened to her?' I finally blurted out as we reached our patient.

'I'm afraid I'm new here,' Sister Claudia replied. 'I hardly know anyone yet by name. Just my young ladies, the cows.'

So that was that, I decided as we reached the young lady she introduced as Gwendolyn.

The cow in front of me was a pitiful sight. Great streams of saliva were hanging from her mouth and she was constantly chomping, as if there was something stuck.

I was startled. The last time I had seen anything like this was during the foot and mouth epidemic. Foot and mouth disease was a disaster for any farmer, but it would be doubly so here on this almost medieval farm where methods had hardly changed in centuries, and where the cows were so loved by the nuns.

Still Practising

Within a few minutes I knew that my fears were groundless. Gwendolyn had no temperature, nothing wrong with her feet and no ulcers on her tongue. But the problem was her tongue. I had seen this particular cow before and remembered her as the most gentle creature, like all the cows on this farm, something surely to do with the gentle way they were treated. Now, however, she chucked her head about this way and that as I tried to get a good look inside her mouth. Eventually I saw that the tongue was very swollen and hard.

The relief that it wasn't foot and mouth freed up some deep memory and suddenly a likely diagnosis came to me, in what felt like a sudden flash of inspiration: wooden tongue, an almost medieval-sounding condition for a medieval farm.

Sister Claudia was still standing quietly beside me, saying nothing. 'I haven't seen this before,' I mused out loud, 'but I think it could be something called wooden tongue.'

But what to do about it. It was caused by a bacterium, as I remembered, something called *Actinobacillus ligniresii*. So in principle an antibiotic would do the trick. But which one? There my memory failed me. Would I ever remember the myriad of bacteria and the diseases they caused? I gave Gwendolyn an injection of penicillin and streptomycin which, once again, something in the lumber room of my brain told me would work, and resolved to come back the next day having got all the answers from Alan.

'Oh, and before you go, I'm afraid we have another patient,' said Sister Claudia just as I was about to be on my way. 'You can probably hear her now.'

From across the covered-in yard, deep in straw, I could hear a plaintive bellowing. My first thought was that it sounded like a cow that had been deprived of her calf. This was usually the case when male – or as the farmers called them 'bobby' – calves were removed from their mothers at four days old to be reared as beef. The mothers often bellowed for days.

But one look at this one told me quite the opposite story. She was exhibiting the classic signs of nymphomania. She had been jumping on or 'riding' the other cows and her back was permanently arched and she had a swollen vulva. It was an easy diagnosis and relatively straightforward treatment. It would probably have been caused by a cystic ovary producing too much female sex hormone. A rectal examination should settle the question, and if I was right, carefully rupturing the cyst through the rectal wall using my fingers would cure the problem.

A minute later with my whole arm in the rectum I could feel the cyst. I was right. I gave a hefty squeeze, and there was a 'pop'. 'There,' I said triumphantly. 'That should cure the problem!'

'What exactly is the problem?' was Sister Claudia's inevitable question.

After a split second of panic I decided upon the blind-'em-with-science approach, not knowing how to broach the subject of nymphomania with a nun.

'Basically it's a follicular problem associated with a relative lack of luteinizing hormone. I have just encouraged ovulation manually.'

'I see,' replied Sister Claudia. 'That's a relief because we thought that she was suffering from nymphomania.'

I related this story to Alan that evening over dinner. He topped it by telling me how when he was a student, a group of them had been taken to see a nymphomaniac cow and when the professor had told them to 'notice her fanny', a

Still Practising

lone female voice had rang out and said, 'What's a fanny?'

Alan had invited me over for dinner in his large country house on the outskirts of town. Although I was on call, no one expected the practice to be busy on the large-animal side that night, and Frank would cope with anything in the small-animal department.

Alan had a lovely rambling house set in a couple of acres of land. A young spaniel puppy called Sweep lolloped around the lounge – seeking attention, with the occasional admonishment to keep him in line. Helen, Alan's wife, was an excellent hostess, always with a twinkle in her eye and taking the mickey out of her husband if he got too serious. He had already quickly briefed me on the treatment for wooden tongue.

My antibiotic treatment had been spot on, it turned out. 'But if you want a quick and permanent solution inject sodium iodide into the vein,' he advised. Not waiting to be asked for more detail he added, 'Ten per cent sodium iodide at a dose of one gram per twenty-five pounds weight.' How did he do it? I'd have to work out for myself how much that would be.

Helen interrupted the conversation. 'Now that's enough. No more shop talk, the poor boy needs some rest. Anyway, what's this about sodium iodide? It's potassium bromide you need!' And with that she gave her husband a playful peck on the cheek.

Helen Jenkins seemed much younger than her years. She was perhaps in her late thirties, pretty and blonde, totally different from my preconceptions of a policewoman, which is what she had been when Alan had met her. And I remembered the WPC who had helped me with the downer cow, the one who hadn't given me a ticket. I hadn't asked Alan or Frank if I could take her out on my rounds. I wasn't

121

sure if I had just forgotten or for once shown a bit of diplomacy. I had never got back to her. However, with Caroline soon off to France . . . I was tempted to ask Alan what were the pitfalls of going out with a policewoman, but he was the boss and I was too much in awe to risk asking personal questions, even though here, in his home environment he was a different person, totally relaxed and enjoying the good life – a million miles from the busy, often stressful life of running a busy practice and keeping young whippersnappers like me in order.

The wine with the meal was delicious; they had brought some bottles back from a recent holiday in Mallorca, Alan said. 'Better than the gut rot you get from the convent,' he laughed. 'I expect you got a bottle today.' I nodded. 'Take my advice,' he continued. 'Leave it in the car for emergency anti-freeze.'

I told him how when I was a student, the landlord at my digs had run an illicit still and produced 80° proof vodka from an assortment of garden produce, including parsnips and potatoes. He charged 5 shillings a bottle. What's more, I said, although it didn't taste of anything, it produced excellent results and was the only drink I'd ever had that consistently failed to deliver a hangover.

I asked Alan about Mallorca and I told him of my slow attempts to learn Spanish. The evening classes Caroline had spotted had folded because there weren't enough takers, so I was still ploughing my way through the *Daily Express* teach-yourself manual. Alan was impressed. He'd never managed much more than *gracias*, he confessed. 'Maybe when I retire,' he said, swirling the wine in his glass, 'which means not for a long time yet.'

His two children, Gary and Suzanne, came in for a goodnight kiss, shepherded by their mother. Both were immaculately behaved and extremely polite. I glanced at the family, the puppy curled up in his basket, the luxurious house. To my young eyes Alan had it all.

I'll have to wait, I thought to myself. I'm only twenty-five.

''E don't like vets, I'm warning yer,' were the first words I heard a week or so later when Mr Adams brought a terrier named Fang in. The unusual fact that I was examining a dog was because Alan and Frank had agreed that I needed more small-animal experience. Of course they were right. Since Nick's arrival nearly nine months before, I had done hardly anything on the domestic front – excluding budgerigars of course, at which I was now considered the practice expert. With Nick due to go on holiday in a few weeks' time, they wanted to make sure I had a good handful of cases to ease myself back in. There were always a mixture of large- and small-animal cases at night, but increasingly I seemed to get the ones that involved a drive – in other words the farm animals – while the senior partner on call got the ones nearer home. I had seen and done so much on the large-animal side over the last couple of years but I still hadn't so much as spayed a cat – very much the bread and butter of small-animal practice.

I knew it was Charles on the phone before he even spoke, by his rasping cough. He was about to go to a sick cow deep in the Weald, approaching Romney Marsh – a good three-quarters of an hour distant. Meanwhile a dog had come in needing a few stitches in its leg. It would need to be given an anaesthetic, otherwise it should be a simple enough job. In any case, he said, Jackie the junior practice nurse was on hand to help me.

The way he said it implied that he didn't think I was up

to it. My own reading was that Charles would far rather I went down to the Weald while he dealt with this particular surgical procedure, and to tell the truth he needed the experience as much as I did. But the senior partners had spoken. I had to build up my experience of small animals, and that was that. As for any difficulties, Jackie and I were good friends; after all I had introduced her to her husband Anthony, Theo's son. We would sort something out.

In fact Anthony was on hand at the surgery when I arrived; he and Jackie were at the stage when they couldn't bear to be parted, so he was usually around when she was on duty. They both came down to help with the wounded dog.

Fang had got into a scrap with a German shepherd and there was a sizeable gash below the elbow. In spite of his name, which I suspected was an attempt at intimidation by his none-too-pleasant owner, the medium-sized, indiscriminate terrier didn't appear too vicious and sat licking the wound on his front leg. I had heard Frank say that it wasn't a good idea to stitch dog bites because they often got infected, but this seemed to be too big a gash to leave to heal by itself.

'Has he been fed?' I asked, looking for a get-out. My attempts at being friendly had been met with a snarl. It had been a long time since I had had anything to do with dogs. The only ones I saw these days were sheep dogs out with shepherds. They are amazing creatures whose loyalty has to be seen to be believed. Get anywhere near their master and they'd have you – much, I thought, like this one. If Fang had eaten recently, any surgery would have to wait till the morning, but no such luck. Apparently he had been 'too choked' after the fight to want his evening meal.

Jackie had already prepared the sedative injection that

Still Practising

would be necessary before giving him the complete anaesthetic. Meanwhile I got a bandage to tie round his nose to stop him biting. And that, I decided was my first priority. I tied a loose knot and proceeded to lasso Fang's nose. The theory was that you would lasso his nose then tie it tight, looping the bandage behind the ears. Once his snout was snapped shut he could snarl as much as he liked, but he wouldn't be able to open his mouth.

Things went wrong almost immediately. I got the noose round his snout but just as I was attempting to tie it behind his ears, with a lightning strike he had got my thumb.

Most dogs would be content to inflict one bite – but Fang was made of a much more vicious disposition. He proceeded to chomp on my thumb as though it were a piece of liver sausage. Seven or eight savage bites (I lost count) followed and try as I might I couldn't get my thumb out of his mouth. I could see the delight in his eyes and hear, above the shouting of his owner, the furious growls as he got to work.

Eventually he let go, and I clutched at the desk with my other hand and sat down, faint with shock and pain. In the corner Fang was cowering under a chair while his owner set about him with a shopping bag. I was in no state to remonstrate and was holding my arm up above my head in an attempt to stop the flow of blood. The bandage that I had planned to secure Fang's snout with was now streaked in red, wrapped round my hand. Within about half a minute, Jackie brought a cup of hot sweet tea for the shock and Frank, who luckily had been at home, arrived in less than ten minutes. Fang immediately met his match; the muzzle was on and he caved in, submitting to the anaesthetic injection like a lamb.

Anthony soon returned, having gone back to the pub to

borrow Theo's car to take me to the hospital for bandaging, antibiotics and a tetanus jab. The pain became a dull throb, sufficient to keep me awake all night.

Frank was on the phone first thing in the morning. I picked it up with my left hand. 'How is it? All swollen up I imagine.'

'Like a banana.'

'Do you think you can drive?'

I hadn't thought about that one. But now that he asked I realized there was no question about it. My right thumb was swollen to twice its size. Not only could I not drive – I couldn't work.

'You'll need at least a week off with that bite,' said Frank, drawing on his own experiences. 'Anyway, that's not your problem. We'll manage. Let us know how things are going in a few days.'

There are times when independence is worth putting on hold, and this was one of them. I packed a few things in a holdall, and Anthony took me to the station where I caught the first train to Rochester. What I needed now was home cooking and recuperation. And there was nothing my mother liked better than ministering to the sick.

Chapter Nine

In some respects Fang's mistaking my thumb for a sausage couldn't have come at a better moment as out of the blue I had been asked by the Amateur Athletics Association if I would run at a meeting at Crystal Palace in July and although I hadn't done any competitive running for nearly a year, I had agreed. An invitation by the AAA is such an honour, I didn't think I could turn it down, but I was sorely unfit. A week of solid practice could make the difference between making a fool of myself and not. So among the things I had thrown in the bag were a pair of running shoes, which was all I needed. The rest, shorts and an old track suit, were still in the wardrobe. My mother never threw anything out. I took it easy at first, but by the end of the week I felt back on form.

The time passed all too quickly and just eight days later I was back in the saddle. The thumb still felt as though it belonged to somebody else, but I could drive. And if a job required the sort of dexterity I couldn't yet manage, I could have help.

My time away had given me space to think. If I couldn't handle nasty bits of work like Fang with ease, not to mention all the routine small-animal work the specialists took for granted, then I couldn't consider myself a proper all-round vet. And I didn't see it getting any better. Was it time to move on? I knew it would be a wrench because I had come to love the practice and the country life. It was certainly something I would have to think about.

In the meantime there was much to enjoy. Caroline had come back for the summer, and was again working at Peggoty's Pantry. She only did lunch times and so by three she was free. One afternoon after work we went off to find the scene of the painting I had bought from Janet Potter. It had been a hot day, too hot, the kind when you never really feel comfortable. But the deep canopy of trees kept everything under it cool and green. I had brought the Ordnance Survey map with me and we parked the car at the pub in a village about 2 miles away that Keith had told me months before was worth a visit. On our walk, following this gurgling stream, we saw nobody – not a soul. When we found the spot, we sat down on the bank by the old bridge and took off our shoes, cooling off our feet in the water. Then we retraced our steps back to the pub for a long drink.

Sometimes Caroline would come out with me on a job – I now kept a spare pair of waders her size in the car. But over everything there was the shadow of the year in France looming, though we rarely talked about it.

The Lightfoots had given up introducing me to unsuitable women – or perhaps they'd given up introducing suitable women to unsuitable me. The friends I met now at their house for dinner were usually couples. Often the Olivers were there, they had become great friends. Sometimes it was just the three of us, when a grateful client gave me some trout, or a rabbit which I immediately passed on to Selina – it wasn't as if I could do anything with them.

Nine months after he arrived in Canterbury, Nick had done what he had set out to do. He was a real small-animal expert now. He had no desire to gain large-animal experience, except for the emergencies he had to undertake like the rest of us. He was entirely single-minded and had recently acquired a dog called Chaos, a King Charles spaniel because, he told me, the breed had a high incidence of heart disease and it would be interesting to study it over a lifetime.

With lambing well and truly over, a lot of my time – at least two days a week – was spent tuberculin testing, having got my Licensed Veterinary Inspector's Certificate the previous summer. Much of the income from a large-animal practice was in working for the Ministry of Agriculture as LVIs, mainly in preventative medicine. The key to this was the eradication of tuberculosis and other diseases such as brucellosis from the national herd.

A tuberculin test works like this. On the first day you go to the herd and each cow has its neck clipped in two places with scissors. Then, after measuring the thickness of the skin, an extract of tuberculin is injected into the bald patches. (Tuberculin is produced from dead and therefore inactivated tuberculosis organisms.)

Three days later you return and measure the thickness of the skin at the injection site. If it is swollen you have a reactor and the cow is culled and examined for the disease. Eventually, so the theory goes, there will be no more reactors. The problem is that thirty years after I was involved in this process, we still haven't eliminated the disease and pockets of infected cows still exist. The current thinking is that badgers are the carriers, but that's another story.

But for me, at the beginning of the seventies, two days a week on a farm doing nothing more strenuous than this was about as good as it got – except when it meant working with Charles who, since the dog-biting episode, seemed to have it in for me.

The AAA meeting was scheduled for a Wednesday afternoon, and I asked to switch my half-day from Friday. Of course I should have had the whole day off. What was I thinking of? But I was naive in those days. I realized my mistake the night before, when I saw I was down to go with Charles to TT test down on the marshes. It was a small farm, with no farm hands, Charles explained, and he needed my help to move the stock. It was the first time this had ever happened and I couldn't help thinking he was being deliberately difficult. But I knew I couldn't leave it any later than twelve if I was to get to Crystal Palace in time. It was hardly ideal preparation, a morning's work, followed by a two-hour drive to arrive half an hour before the race.

At about 11.30 we were nearly finished and I was breathing a sigh of relief when Charles took the wind out of my sails. 'Just before you shoot off, David, there are a couple of things to do up in Thanet.'

'Look,' I said, 'I'm off this afternoon, as you know. And I have to drive to London. I just can't do it, Charles.' At least, I thought with relief, we had taken two cars.

Charles didn't hide his displeasure and without another word, turned on his heel.

I got to Crystal Palace with less than forty-five minutes to spare, having driven as fast as I dared, and went straight to the dressing room where the first person I saw was Jeffrey Archer.

We had run against each other several times before when I was captain of London University and he was President of the Oxford Union. On each occasion we had done the same time, but each time he had come first and I had come second.

Jeffrey Archer was already a celebrity, although at that time he hadn't written a book, or become an MP, or campaigned to be London's mayor. He was very sure of himself, though, and I remembered him as being very competitive – very much more so than me. That afternoon, as we were changing, I saw him going through the running order to check who he would be running against, and saw it was me. He looked up, took in the AAA shirt (to wear a AAA vest is on a par with running for England), gave a sniff, and turned away. I knew he was just doing it to psych me out. It was normal practice to try and psych your opponents out – I used to do it myself to athletes I considered myself better than. But even so, it riled me. So perhaps it worked, because although I made a good start and was beating him, I felt him draw level and just pip me on the line. Just like all the races we had had – some half a dozen in all.

On balance I hadn't done too badly, given my lack of preparation. On the way back to Canterbury when the meeting was over, I was cursing Charles for putting a spanner in the works but it was my fault really. All I could think of was this profession of mine and everything else had to come second. Even running for the AAA was not terribly important – important enough that I decided do it, but not important enough to think before booking myself in for a morning's work. If you are going to run against people like Jeffrey Archer and be under scrutiny by the England selectors, you do not traipse around a farm in the morning, then drive two hours up to Crystal Palace, then get straight into your track suit and run. But this is how stupid I was. And I really had thought it would be all right.

'But that's brilliant,' said Caroline when I told her. 'You came second, that's amazing.' But she didn't understand. In athletics coming second doesn't count. It's all about winning, as Jeffrey Archer knows only too well.

The sky that I could see through the latticework of green which in high summer made tunnels of the narrow lanes was bright blue, with the promise of a lovely day ahead as Jackie and I drove to Jed Dickens' farm in the Weald. Jed's herd was up to 100 cows and the curmudgeonly old so-and-so who had given me such a rough time when I had first arrived in the practice had almost overnight become the most amiable fellow you could wish to meet. The reason? After years on his own, he'd remarried, a quiet widow from the next village he'd known all his life.

'When I think of all those wasted years, David,' he said. 'And all the time she were no more'n a walk away.'

Because a TT test is pretty much routine, there was plenty of scope for good hearted banter and gossip as we got the cows in. Each one had to be persuaded to enter the stocks that we used to restrain them. A bar would come down round the neck while someone – in this case Jed – held the head still. Each cow had to be identified by breed and ear-tag number. Then I would clip the neck, measure the skin thickness and call out the measurement, which Jackie would write down.

Halfway through the morning, we stopped for a break and Jed disappeared into the kitchen, returning with a flagon of beer and three pint glasses. Sitting on a low brick wall in front of the house, in the shade of a cherry tree, sipping the local ale was my idea of heaven. Over the other side of the barnyard we watched as two geese and a cockerel squabbled over a crust of bread the new Mrs Dickens had just thrown out.

Suddenly I was overcome by an enormous sneeze, followed by three more in succession.

'Well, that's a turn up, David. Allergic to beer now are you?' Jed chortled. It had been my ability to handle my beer that changed Jed's opinion of the 'townie greenhorn'.

I joined in the laughter. But later, with my eyes closed, in the soporific state induced by the sunshine and the good Kentish ale, it set me thinking. I'd been doing a lot of sneezing lately, particularly when I was TT testing I realized, and particularly on the first day when I had to clip the necks. On the second visit, when I had to read the test, it wasn't so bad.

'You're burning the candle at both ends, that's your trouble,' observed Jed when we were about to leave. 'You should see your eyes, they're bright red!'

'Are they, Jackie?' I asked when we were on our way back. She said she hadn't noticed.

I took a quick glance in the rearview mirror. It was true. My eyes were definitely pink and sore, and I had a terrible itch in my throat. A paroxysm of sneezing seized me as I drew into the hospital car park.

Frank was on his way out to a meeting in London. 'Hay fever,' he said without hesitation after a quick glance. 'You need some antihistamines.' Then he hesitated. 'Bit late for it though – August. The grass pollen season begins in June and ends in July.'

Trust him to know the seasons for grass pollination. Typical – you could ask a hundred vets and they wouldn't know, but Frank was a mine of information on just about anything. I wondered if he had ever come across allergy to cows – because that's what I was beginning to think I had. There was no chance to ask him as he shot out of the car park in his brand new Citroën – a beautiful car with all the latest comforts.

I resolved to be a bit more scientific about these bouts of sneezing and runny eyes, and to make a note when I had them. Maybe I should see a doctor too – it was starting to make tuberculin testing a chore. It was a shame: I did so love being on a farm all day chatting away to the farmers and their families doing something which wasn't too difficult or stressful.

David Grant

The other fount of all knowledge was Keith, although his area of expertise was rather different from Frank's. Pubs, beer and women were his special subjects. I bumped into him later in the Spotted Cow. Jenny had let him out for the evening, he said. Over a pint I told him my suspicions about the cows.

'Just as well it isn't human females,' he said and spluttered into his beer at the thought of it. 'Talking of which, how's the copper's daughter coming along?'

'Off to France for a year next month,' I said, gloomily.

'You'll be laughing if it's Calais.'

'Toulouse' I said.

'Then you'd better be careful not Toulouse her!'

His joke barely raised a smile. 'Do you realize Keith, I don't even know where it is.'

'Don't say you haven't talked about it.'

'Not much,' I admitted ruefully.

'It's where they make Concorde isn't it? Somewhere in the south maybe. Long way from here, anyway,' he added as he got up to get another pint in.

It was all right for Keith. He had fixed his wedding with Jenny for early September. Jackie and Anthony had married in May. I sighed. Everybody was getting married except me. It struck me sometimes that I was like two different people: one feeling sorry for myself because I was not getting married, the other in total panic at the idea. But how could I marry on the sort of money I earned? Keith earned twice as much as I did. I knew it would be worth it in time, but how long? Although I had become much more confident with farm practice over the last few months, my thoughts turned increasingly to my need to do some small-animal work. I knew nothing about surgery. The niggle that began when I was recuperating from the dog bite had started up again. I knew I would have to move if I wanted extensive small-animal experience. Nick was in the middle of his own learning curve and showed no sign of leaving.

'Never mind, me old mate,' said Keith as he returned from the bar. 'There'll be a new crop of students in the house next month, and I can see you now with your tongue hanging out.'

I laughed out loud. Mrs Nightingale had told me that there going to be twelve girls coming in September, all first-years at the local teacher training college. 'The last lot looked about fourteen. They seem to get younger and younger – or am I getting old?' I peered at myself in the mirror behind the bar as I got the next round in. The red eyes certainly didn't help.

Just then Theo's wife, Maureen, came down from upstairs. 'You look rough David! Too many late nights. They been getting you out of bed?'

'I have had a rough few weeks,' I replied, deciding not to mention the allergy, but Keith got in first.

'Would you believe it? The Cisco Kid is allergic to cows!'

This caused great amusement and I would be ribbed about it for evermore. Perhaps it was something my system would get used to, I rationalized. On the other hand perhaps it would get worse, like bee stings. At any rate I would have to work out what part of the cow I was allergic to, I decided. As things turned out I was going to get plenty of opportunity over the next couple of weeks.

About ten days later I found myself on Bob Adams' farm. Three cows had aborted on the same day. This had all the hallmarks of a complete disaster. Bob had a huge farm, one of the earliest really to go for intensive milk production. Everything was the very latest in technology. The only thing lacking was the sophisticated computers of today. With getting on for 400 cows on the farm an abortion storm, as it was called, was the very last thing that anyone wanted.

Normally Alan or Charles would have been come but they were both away on a course, so Frank sent me to do some preliminary work. He gave me one of his potted seminars on what he suspected might be the cause of the abortions: brucellosis, a very nasty disease to get in a dairy herd. It would cause late abortions and spread to the other cows. Likely as not the afterbirth would not come away properly and so cause an infection of the womb. Infertility would result and the economic effects of this on a large enterprise didn't bear thinking about.

My instructions were to get some samples of the afterbirth and take blood samples to send off to the Ministry laboratories. 'Make sure you stay as sterile as possible,' was Frank's parting shot. The last thing I wanted was to get the disease myself. The effects of this were just becoming apparent in vets, many of whom had contracted it by germs entering cuts in the skin. The effects were debilitating – everything from crippling arthritis to an intermittent fever causing flu-like symptoms.

So masked up with plastic aprons and gloves on every conceivable part of my body I did as I was told. If it did turn out to be brucellosis, the rescue plan would be up to Alan.

A month later I was back at Bob Adams' place again, to do a TT test for the herd. In the end, twenty of his cows had aborted and had been disposed of, while all the young stock were being vaccinated and strict hygienic measures were in place. I had spent hours on the farm over the last few weeks vaccinating all the susceptible animals, and it looked as if the worst was over. Bob had lost the worried frown he had developed since the abortions began. Although it was a big financial setback at least he didn't face ruin. The Bob that turned out to help me with the tuberculin test was like a different person. Jackie was with me again, and on the way down I had to stop the car because she felt sick. I gave her a look, and she admitted that he was pregnant, though she asked me not to say anything at the practice yet.

I had been on Bob's farm on numerous occasions over the last few weeks without a hint of trouble. But within minutes of clipping the cows' necks the sneezing started. After an hour it was becoming more than a joke. At least I knew now what was causing the allergy – it was the hair. Stopping for a cup of tea I rummaged around in the boot of the car for the mask which I had used extensively to protect myself from brucellosis. Even that didn't seem to help as the tiny particles of hair still irritated my eyes. By the end of the day I was a sorry sight, with puffed up eyelids and red eyes.

There was no need to see a doctor. I knew what the diagnosis would be – I was allergic to cow dander. I just had to avoid it. But what did that mean for a large-animal vet? There was only one sensible answer. But I decided not to say anything to the partners until I had a definite plan.

A few weeks later I was browsing through the *Veterinary Record*, the vets' professional journal. It comes out weekly and is less formal than it sounds, with a mixture of interesting articles, news items, marriages, births and deaths, and in those days a few pages of job adverts.

Nowadays there is a glut of jobs but then each job was keenly contested. For me it was just a matter of time until something caught my eye. I had been looking carefully for a couple of weeks when I saw a big box advert offering a job in one of the newest small-animal hospitals in the country. The Sir Harold Harmsworth Memorial Animal Hospital was in inner London and run by the RSPCA. I

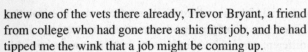

David Grant

knew one of the vets there already, Trevor Bryant, a friend from college who had gone there as his first job, and he had tipped me the wink that a job might be coming up.

In London it would be a lot easier to study Spanish, I thought. There were sure to be plenty of language schools, as I had outgrown my *Daily Express* course. And on the career front it was an ideal environment to cover the widest possible range of small animal surgery and, who knows, in a few years I could return to the country in a mixed practice. Only one night a week on call, it had said in the advertisement, and four out of five weekends off. I might even take up my athletic career again! It sounded too good to be true.

I began to plan my life. Caroline would be back in a year following her year in France and I would be able to see her all the time. Her college was only two miles away from the hospital. The whole thing began to look more and more attractive. I wrote in for an application form and a couple of weeks later I found myself on the train to London having been short-listed for interview.

To prepare myself and to seem keen, I had done my best to find out something about Sir Harold. He had died tragically young, at the age of only 55. A philanthropist and an animal lover he wanted to have a hospital built in London so that the poor in the area who couldn't afford private vets could get the best possible treatment according to their means. At the time of his death he was the owner of *The Field* magazine.

The hospital had been opened only three years before and stood like an oasis on undeveloped waste land, although I wasn't to find that out until later. The interview was conducted in the headquarters in Jermyn Street, an old windy building in which you could get lost very easily. The appointments panel consisted of the Chief Vet of the hospital,

138

Tony Self, the Personnel Manager and the Chief Vet of the society. I got a good grilling, far worse than I expected. The great disadvatage, of course, was that I could offer very little small-animal experience. A plus was the fact that I had been working in one of the best animal hospitals in the country. And I was honest with them – even though I knew little about small animals I would give it my best shot.

After some muttering amongst themselves, Tony Self came over to me and said they were interested. Would I like to have a look at the hospital to 'see what's on offer and we can discuss it further?'

So there and then, he and I left the building and took the Piccadilly Line to Finsbury Park. From there it was a five-minute walk. The hospital was certainly impressive, and enormous compared to the one at Canterbury. The wards were full of all manner of dogs and cats, and other animals that I hadn't expected – two hedgehogs I remember, even wild birds.

There were two spanking new operating theatres – one even had closed-circuit television and a preparation room which was a hive of bustle and energy when we passed through. But the clincher was what lay above the hospital – a flat. None of the other vets had need of it, he said. 'How would £2,200 plus the flat sound?'

'Done!' I replied. I didn't tell him that I would have worked for £500 less. I would have to buy my own car, but the flat made up for that. And anyway, it wasn't as if I would have far to travel to work – four flights of stairs to be precise. I was suddenly overwhelmed by the excitement of it all. I hadn't even asked about the on-call rota but even that was a bonus. Only one night a week and one weekend in five with the others off. I was on cloud nine.

Chapter Ten

Only when the train pulled into the station back at Canterbury did the adrenalin rush of the new job give way to the reality of just what I was leaving. Three years is a long time. There were my friends; Keith in particular had become part of my life, though it must be said that since Jenny had stolen his heart the nights out with the lads had been fewer and further between. But a life that didn't revolve around a nightly visit to the Spotted Cow to be entertained with Theo's brand of landlord humour mitigated by exceptionally well-kept beer would be hard to imagine. At least there I wouldn't be forgotten: it was me, after all, who had introduced Theo's son Anthony to Jackie, his wife. Soon Theo and Maureen would be grandparents. And as for the Mrs Nightingale – well after nearly three years as her tenant, in many ways she was as good as family.

As I got out of the car back at the house, she gave me a cheery wave as she took in the washing on the line, sheet after flapping sheet. It was the last week before her students left for the summer. I gave her a cheery wave back. How was I going to tell her? Although the atmosphere had been difficult after I split up with Angie things had improved considerably when Angie herself had moved out, and that was a year ago now. The problem was that Mrs Nightingale had thought we were made for each other. I knew because she had told me often enough. Even after Angie had left and it was no longer a question of loyalties, if ever she saw me looking gloomy she'd say, 'Well, David, you've only got yourself to blame,' and the dangly earrings that she favoured would wobble as she shook her head.

Mrs Nightingale had even come round to accepting Caroline, though she never said anything directly. Perhaps she had decided it was wisest to stay out of my love life.

Now she had other things on her mind, counting the days until the latest little Nightingale arrived on the scene. Phil lived in Richmond, in west London, but Mrs Nightingale was planning to go over there as soon as the baby was born and help out for a few weeks. As an airline pilot Phil couldn't hope to be around as much as he would like, and his wife Sue's own mother had died when she was only a teenager. Fortunately Mrs Nightingale had so much else going on in her life that she never imposed herself, but she was a natural mother to whoever needed mothering at the time, and that of course had included Angie, which is why things had been so strained between us.

At least after Angie I hadn't got involved with any other of Mrs Nightingale's 'young charges', as she liked to call them. And they seemed to be getting younger, I thought, as I walked to my door. From the attic I could hear what I had been reliably informed was a group called Slade blasting out. Slade? Call that music? I harumphed to myself as I put the key in the lock of the garden flat. Whatever happened to real music, the Beatles, Donovan, Cat Stevens, the Kinks? There was no doubt about it, I was definitely growing old: I was beginning to sound like my father.

A tin of baked beans was quickly opened and while I was waiting for it to heat through, I trawled through my record collection for something that would match my mood and chose Beethoven's Pastoral Symphony. I sat down on

David Grant

the settee, closed my eyes and inevitably my thoughts
strayed to all the girls who had shared it with me: Sally,
Chantal, Julia, Angie. Even Caroline. I sighed. Suddenly a
smell of scorched tomato sauce broke my reverie. I jumped
up and promptly caught my leg on the corner of what passed
for a dining table in this tiny flat, where nothing was
more than two feet apart. At least that wouldn't happen
in the acres of space that awaited me in the flat above
the Harmsworth, I thought, as I hopped painfully through to
the kitchen.

The worst part was going to be telling the bosses. Even
though I would be giving them two months' notice, it
wasn't a cosy prospect. How should I do it? Over the last
three years I'd become quite good at breaking bad news to
pet owners. I usually managed a 'good news, bad news'
approach, as in 'Well Fido has obviously had a happy life
and the pain/suffering will soon be over.' But however
many times I tried the words of my resignation out, nothing
seemed right. And there was the question of protocol.
Should I tell Alan first – as the senior large-animal vet he
would be what we would call today my 'line manager'?
Best would be to get both Frank and Alan together, I
decided, although my heart sank at the thought of it. If only
I could just write an 'FA/AJ to see DG' note in the diary.

'What's up David?' Frank said as he came into the
library the next morning, resplendent in a red and white
spotted bow tie. I would miss those, I thought. 'You look as
though you lost a pound and found a penny. Not another
love affair gone wrong?'

I swallowed. This was the moment. And earlier than
I had expected. 'Not exactly, I said, 'though in some
ways . . .' then I faltered.

Frank had the antennae of a short wave wireless set and

142

immediately sensed I was serious. He pulled a couple of chairs out from the table and motioned me to sit down, his forehead pulled into a physical manifestation of a question mark. 'Go on.'

'I don't know how to say this,' I began.

'You're leaving.'

I felt a weight lifting from me as his words echoed round the high-ceilinged room. I nodded.

'Well.' There was just a slight pause before he went on, 'Best part of three years you've been with us now, David. So I can't say I'm surprised, particularly in the light of this allergy business. And I know you haven't had the small-animal experience you might have wanted.'

For the first time I had the courage to raise my head look him in the eye. 'I can't help feeling that I'm letting you down, all you've done for me.'

'Nonsense. You've proved yourself a highly valued member of the team. No, David. Looking at it dispassionately, you're doing exactly the right thing, though of course we'll be very sorry to lose you.'

He began to tidy the handful of periodicals on the table into a neat pile.

'Got something else lined up I take it?'

'Er, yes. The RSPCA. Their new hospital in north London. The Harmsworth Memorial Hospital.'

'Indeed.' Frank nodded. 'Well, I've heard good things about it and you'll certainly get enough small-animal experience there. And not much contact with cow dander,' he laughed.

I laughed too, though more with relief than at the rather weak joke.

'You haven't told Alan yet, I take it,' he continued.

'No, I was hoping to tell you together, but, well . . .'

143

'Yes, yes, of course. You won't mind if I tell him myself will you? We're meeting at the solicitors later this morning, some partnership business. So, if you don't mind?'

I carried on with the day's visits, one of which was Roy Gibbons. 'What's up, David?' he said, as I joined him and Katharine for a cup of tea and home-made shortbread dipped in chocolate. A good thing I wasn't a criminal, I thought, it seemed I couldn't hide anything from anyone.

As usual the Gibbonses were wonderful and fully understood why I had to go and, as committed Christians, managed to make me feel that working for the RSPCA – helping animals and the poor at the same time – I was next to St Francis in their estimation.

They say you never really appreciate something until it's gone, and it really did seem that I was more appreciated than I thought. It was a story that would be repeated again and again over the next few days. Talking over old times, funny incidents – and I'd had more than my fair share of those – made me begin to wonder if I was doing the right thing. Roy and Katharine's view, it soon transpired, was not shared by anyone else; the opinion generally among my farmer clients was that I was mad to be leaving the beauties of Kent for a derelict bomb site in that hotbed of sin and iniquity, London.

It was now high summer and the long grass bordering the lanes and byways that my trusty old Anglia took me down that afternoon was just beginning to take on a bleached look. The hedgerows that had for so long been a uniform green had begun to separate out, the colours of the different plants subtly changing, making a patchwork of greens and golds. Between them heads of red and white campion nodded as the car passed by. In shadier areas fox-gloves grew taller and taller as the lower flowers shrivelled and dropped, just like the hollyhocks that lined the paths of village cottages, some of them taller than me. Now that I knew I was leaving, it was as if I saw everything more clearly, like the Polaroid sunglasses that I had bought that summer.

Like the gentleman he was, Alan made it easy for me. I must have arrived back at the hospital just a few minutes after he did – I hardly had time to register his car before he walked towards me beaming. He was wearing a sprig of honeysuckle in his buttonhole, I noticed. I wouldn't meet his like again either.

'Congratulations, David. Wonderful news. Though that's not to say we won't miss you. The garage definitely will,' I laughed at this sideways swipe at my accident track record. 'Just what you needed I should say. No more irascible farmers eh? Not to mention irascible colleagues.'

Nick was his usual effervescent self. He said I was to keep a record of all the heart cases I came across, though he slightly fazed me by asking me how long I planned to stay at the Harmsworth and what I planned to do afterwards. Afterwards? I hadn't even walked through the doors of the place.

Telling Caroline wasn't a problem: in fact she was delighted. Like me, she saw the long-term advantages: Harmsworth was so close to her college and, when I'd told her I planned to return to athletics, she giggled. 'All that running around will keep you out of trouble!' I didn't even flinch – I was getting better at 'commitment'. Not that I said anything in particular, it was more that I happily listened to her talking about next year and how great it would be, the two of us in London. It gave us a certain parity somehow, and suddenly she was talking about Toulouse, a subject we never discussed. It was nice to see her all fired up and excited. It wasn't like today when nearly everyone has been abroad. Like me she had been on a school exchange, but that was it. France seemed much more foreign than it does today, when all you do is arrive at Waterloo with a credit card; it would take her more than twenty-four hours to get there. But she was coming back for Christmas, and I would go out for Easter. I planned to drive down and we'd explore the Tarn gorges and the lower Pyrenees. I'd already asked Dad to look out for a car for me.

The moment that was really hard was when I saw my job advertised the following week in the *Veterinary Record*. I suddenly had a serious attack of butterfly tummy and spent an evening going over it with Keith, aided by a few pints. Though frankly he wasn't much help: with his forthcoming marriage to Jenny only three weeks away, he was as jittery as I was. It was all we could do to prop each other up.

But for both of us the die was cast and the remaining weeks flew by in a strange mixture of nostalgia and anticipation; nothing really seemed very real.

Caroline and I went up to Liverpool for the wedding, which was everything you could expect, with half the male guests Everton fans, and the rest Tottenham supporters. Keith was resplendent in an outfit that owed more to Rod Stewart than Moss Bros, and Jenny looked sensational in a traditional white dress. She had been planning to wear something short, but it was Selina who had pointed out that fashions change but wedding photographs stay on the mantelpiece for ever. A good piece of advice.

Caroline and I then went on to the Lake District for a long weekend. We rented a cottage, bought proper walking boots in Keswick, and a supply of Kendal Mint Cake. With our brightly coloured cagoules and red socks, and a map in a plastic folder on a string, we looked just like professional fellwalkers. I soon discovered that the Lake District has more than its fair share of excellent country pubs, which were pleasurable destinations.

We hadn't spent this long together since Christmas, and yet we both felt completely comfortable. We even seemed to enjoy walking at the same pace. The weather was kind to us: blue skies and yet never too hot to be uncomfortable. The last day, after a walk to Buttermere, Caroline got quite weepy, but it was more about leaving England than anything to do with me; there was less than a week to go before she was due in Toulouse. Back in Canterbury we had a final meal with Nick and Selina that Caroline said she didn't believe could be surpassed anywhere in France: roast chicken cooked in butter and lemon juice served with rice washed down with two bottles of Sancerre. Although we were all very cheery, there was an unstated sadness in the air. This was our last supper, both in the real sense and metaphorically speaking. Luckily for me it was far from my last supper cooked by Selina, although the next one was a good few years away, when we caught up with each other again in Edinburgh.

Two days later I turned up at the Hitchenses' house, and waited in the car while Caroline said tearful farewells to her mother – Ken was on duty, which was why my services as chauffeur had been accepted. Then I drove her down the wonderful old Roman road towards Dover. We were both quiet, Caroline thinking of the country she was leaving behind, me thinking that I might never take this only too familiar road again. She had a long journey in front of her: ferry, train to Paris, then change from the Gare du Nord to the Gare St Lazare. We had talked about my going as far as Paris with her, but as I only had another week to go myself, it just wasn't practical. Charles Harte was away on holiday and the practice couldn't manage without two large-animal vets.

Ever since I had told Mrs Nightingale I was leaving, she had treated me like a prodigal son. Slices of cake and offers of tea or coffee, not to mention joining the family for supper, became a regular hazard as I returned to the flat after work. The students were away on their summer holidays and she missed the company, I think, although the arrival of young Toby had caused great excitement, and photographs of a bald baby held by the doting grandmother were in pride of place on the kitchen dresser. Only once did she ask me about my successor but there was nothing I could tell her apart from his name. I surprised myself, however, by feeling more than a twinge of jealousy at this young man who would supplant me in her affections.

Before I knew it, I was packing my things. It's surprising how much stuff you accumulate over three years, and a few days before actually leaving, I drove home to Rochester in the Anglia with a car-load.

On my last day I left as I had wanted – quietly, with no fuss. I'd had a drink with Barbara, the head practice nurse, and Pauline at the Spotted Cow the previous night and I'd already said goodbye to Charles ten days before, as he was due to return the day I started at the Harmsworth. Charles and I had had our disagreements, but to be fair he was a first-class clinician and I had never forgotten the help he had given me in those first anxious six months.

Keith was still away on honeymoon but there was talk of him getting an area manager's job with the snack company that he worked for, so I would doubtless be seeing him in London, I thought.

After saying my goodbyes to Mrs Nightingale – goodbyes that had already lasted for several weeks – I gave the flat a final check, then with a sigh locked the door for the last time and walked round to the hospital with the couple of suitcases that were left. I said goodbye to my colleagues, Barbara's eyes were distinctly moist, and for the first time I felt choked myself. I forgot to say thanks to Frank for all that he in particular had done for me. I am grateful that I was able to do so many years later when our paths crossed again.

I had been let off evening surgery and Alan, my old friend and mentor, drove me to the station to get the train to Rochester. We swung round to the east side of town to get to the station. Alan was thoughtful in the car and didn't say much. Maybe he felt as I often do now when a colleague I have been working with day in and day out for a couple of years moves on. Sometimes you may never see them again for years – people, friends, you've shared a life with – and even then it might be nothing more than bumping into them at a congress. But I was about to enter a world of small-animal medicine and surgery, and Alan was firmly fixed in the world of farm animals. Our paths probably wouldn't cross again.

As the train pulled in we shook hands. 'Good luck,' Alan said. 'And thanks. It's been a pleasure seeing you develop into a valued colleague.' I could sense that he was genuinely sad to see me go. A mini-wave of panic engulfed me. Was I doing the right thing in leaving? I got into the carriage. It was too late now.

There was that moment of hiatus, when goodbyes have been said and there's nothing more to do except wait for the train to go. Then the whistle went and the last doors were shut and we began to move. 'Thanks for everything,' I shouted over the noise. 'I'll keep in touch.'

My mood lightened as the train sped through the countryside. London was only a couple of hours away after all and I could come back to Canterbury whenever I wanted. But things never turn out quite as you expect. Soon I would be enveloped in another way of life, far more frenetic, and, as things turned out, I never saw Alan again. He was to suffer a fatal heart attack in his early sixties and his loss left me immensely saddened.

From Canterbury to Rochester is not far, but that evening I felt as emigrants must have felt when they left for Australia or America – as if, whatever happened next for better or for worse, this chapter of my life was over, something that belonged to the past, never to be revisited. And in many ways it never was. I sat with my back to the engine watching as Kentish orchards with their doll's house trees and hop gardens still heavy with green vines receded into the fast-fading horizon, all too soon making way for the paint factories of the Medway valley, the other Kent, the other England.

My father met me at Rochester station in his pride and joy, a two-tone Morris Oxford. He was looking particularly pleased with himself as he'd found a car for me. He had been on the case since he heard about the job and this was perfect, he said, ten years old, only 10,000 on the clock. A Riley 1.5, it had belonged to the father of a friend of his who had died of a stroke a month or so back. Now the friend wanted it to go to a good home. It was in beautiful condition and only £50.

I had fond memories of the Riley 1.5 as the vet in Rochester where I had helped out from the age of fifteen had had an identical one. It seemed like only last year, but with a shock I realized that over ten years had passed since those days; my memories were as old as the car.

Dad took me to see it next morning and he was right, it was a beauty, immaculate inside and out, with leather seats but no radio. After a trip to Halfords, and with Dad's expertise with all things electrical, that was soon remedied.

The next day my mother had prepared a big Sunday lunch, though it felt a bit strange eating roast pork and apple sauce with the thermometer outside the kitchen window reading well over 70 degrees. It was a birthday tradition that dated from when I was about eight, when the crackling on roast pork was my favourite food. In fact my birthday was the following day, which seemed very appropriate with what felt like a whole new chapter of my life about to begin.

I left as soon as lunch was over, the car piled high with everything I thought I would need. When I had heard I'd got the job I had telephoned Trevor to give him the good news and he'd told me that the flat had everything I would need. It had never been offered to him, because by the time he took the job at the Harmsworth, he was already married; he lived with his wife Susannah, a teacher, in Muswell Hill out to the north, in a big old rambling house which needed everything done to it. All I needed to take, he said, were a few personal items. But it still added up: two suitcases of clothes, one of Janet Potter's pictures, my record player and ever-growing collection of records, two boxes of books, a few tins of soup and baked beans and a half-empty jar of Nescafé left over from Canterbury, and a screw-top jam jar of milk that Mum handed to me just as I was leaving.

'But I can get some in London,' I told her. In answer she just pursed her lips. She wasn't convinced, even though I hadn't let on just how desolate the area I was moving to was. 'Near Hampstead' was how I had described it to her with a little poetic licence. And it was, geographically speaking. The Harmsworth was not far from the Holloway Road, and Holloway was just across the heath, but in every other way it was like the East End: run down and generally unloved. The catchment area for the Harmsworth was enormous, anywhere north of the Thames and east of Hampstead. The hospital itself was just off the A1, one of the pollution-clogged arterial routes leading out of London. Getting there was simple – I just followed signs saying 'Cambridge and the North'.

I parked the Riley and got out. The air was dusty, as only London can be after a hot summer's day. The rough ground around the hospital was bright with rosebay willowherb, the pinkish red flowers that, together with ragwort, seemed to be the only thing that grew on the wasteland. Inside the hospital sat a few people – emergencies. I went across to reception.

A young nurse smiled at me. 'Name?'

'David Grant. I wonder—'

'Ah yes. You phoned about the parrot.'

'No, I—'

'It's in the exotics ward. If you wouldn't mind waiting a few minutes, I'll take you round. Did you bring a cage?'

'No, I . . .'

'No? Well, I'm sorry but I really don't think that I can release him to you. I suggest you come back tomorrow with the cage. You needn't worry, he's quite happy here,' at which she flashed me a lovely smile.

'Look, I'm sorry . . .' I began.

'No need to be sorry. These things happen, Mr Grant, but like I said, he's quite safe where he is.'

'But I don't have a parrot,' I finally managed to blurt out.

'Then why did you say on the phone that you did?' the girl said, looking at me as if I boasted pointed ears like *Star Trek*'s Mr Spock.

'But I didn't. It wasn't me. It must have been somebody

else. I was told to come to reception to collect the keys to the upstairs flat. I am the new vet.'

Just then we both turned at the sound of metal scraping on glass as a man with a face dominated by a red beard struggled to open the heavy glass door while carrying a bird cage the size of a fridge.

'I've come about my parrot,' he said. 'I spoke to you earlier, you said you were holding an African grey that had been found on Hampstead Heath. Name's Grant.'

The flat was reached either by an outside door that opened onto a staircase, or through the hospital itself. Gill, as I soon discovered the young nurse was called, phoned up to the nurses' common room to get another nurse to stand in for her while she took me up herself. The flat was even bigger than I had imagined. It had two double bedrooms, and a sitting room that was bigger than Mrs Nightingale's. The windows looked west towards Hampstead and the sun was streaming in, filling the flat with light. I could hardly believe my luck and just wished I could call Caroline and tell her what she had to look forward to. But she was in Toulouse and I didn't even have a telephone number.

But the thought reminded me to call my mother. I picked up the phone. No dialling tone, just silence. Then a man's voice. 'Yes?'

'Oh. I – is that the switchboard?'

'Ah, you must be the new vet.'

'Yes. I wanted to make a phone call.'

'No problem. I'll get you a line. My name's Andy by the way. On the first floor, right underneath you. Drop in and say hello when you're ready. I'm here all night.'

No direct line. Hmmm. I supposed I should have to get my own phone installed.

It took four trips up four flights of stairs to empty the

Riley of my worldly possessions, then I drove it around the back. With Janet's picture on the wall and my books on the bookcase and the record player plugged in, I decided to have a cup of celebratory coffee. The kitchen was like an advertisement, fitted units and the kind of flooring they used in Flash television commercials, even an electric toaster. What more could a man want? Then I knew. Sugar. In those days the idea of coffee without sugar was more than I could bear.

I picked up the phone again. 'Andy?'

'Yes David. Another line?'

'No. Look, I don't suppose you have any sugar do you?'

We both laughed. It was the standard excuse from the script of every sit-com that has ever been written.

The quickest way to get to their room, Andy said, was down the fire escape. 'It's that door straight across the landing, you can't miss it.'

Sure enough, like something out of *The Lion, the Witch and the Wardrobe*, I opened the door and there was a metal ladder with rungs about two feet wide leading down to the floor below. Gingerly I stepped down and at the bottom found another door which led to the corridor. The night room was directly opposite. I knocked on the door. It was opened by a man in his mid forties, with short, nearly crew-cut hair going grey. The most striking thing about him were his eyes which were a startling china blue. 'Hi. Come in.'

The room was directly below the smaller of my two bedrooms. On one side were two bunk beds, on the other a long desk with two telephones. Beside the desk, on top of a small fridge, was a kettle, a large tin of Nescafé and a bag of sugar on a small tray that could have done with a clean. The sink was piled high with mugs. Andy took one, gave it a quick swill under the tap, dried it, then filled it with sugar.

Just then one of the phones went. He sat down at the desk. 'Harmsworth Memorial Hospital.' There was a pause while he motioned me to sit down as well. As the conversation on the phone continued I idly picked up a book from the pile on the desk. Voltaire: *Candide*. Hmmm. And another one, *Montaigne's Essays*. Not exactly Agatha Christie.

Andy put the phone down. 'Nothing that can't wait till tomorrow,' he said, by way of explanation. 'Limping cat. Been limping for a couple of weeks. We get a lot of that here.'

Andy was one of the small team of drivers as they were called, who were in charge of the phone calls at night. They would drive out and collect any animals which were seriously ill for the duty vet to deal with if they thought that was necessary. Many of these calls were the results of RTAs, as I learned to call them later – road traffic accidents. Andy and his colleagues, Bill and Roy, weren't trained in any formal way but over the years they had built up a knowledge that was invaluable – and not just about animals.

'Yea,' he said as he saw me looking at the books. 'I'm into French seventeenth century philosophy at the moment. You know, *amour propre*.'

Mystified, I ransacked what passed for my French vocabulary. '*Amour*' rang a definite bell, but '*propre*'? Proper? Clean?

'Self-esteem,' he said in response to my puzzled look.

I nodded. I later learned that Andy had just missed going to university because of the war. He did his training in the army but by the time he had finished it was all over. He'd worked for a local newspaper in Yorkshire but hated the lifestyle, with its drinking and 'vulture mentality' as he called it. Then in the early sixties he had gone to India –

long before the Beatles had made it fashionable. It was there he had become interested in philosophy and religions. He and his wife, whom he'd met in India, had come back a few years ago and he was driving for a wine company when he heard about this job. He'd become interested in the Jains in India, the sect that don't believe in killing even an ant, which in turn had made him interested in animals generally – the philosophy of animals, rather than the nitty-gritty stuff that vets did, he explained.

He lived with his wife Ellen in a flat in Islington, where she was a social worker. It was only ten minutes' walk away and this job gave him the opportunity to read in peace and to exercise control, he explained. I saw what he meant a few minutes later when the phone rang again. 'Harmsworth Memorial Hospital.' Long pause. 'I suggest you take him to your nearest vet in the morning. If you tell me where you live, I'll give you an address and telephone number.'

Even from where I was sitting I could hear the raised voice at the other end.

'Are you a pensioner or unemployed?' He took the phone away from his ear as the barrage continued. 'Look friend,' he said, 'I don't know what time you got up this morning, but I've been up since seven. I suggest you make yourself a cup of tea and contact your local vet in the morning.' And he put the phone down. People often assumed that as long as they rang outside ordinary hours they could get free treatment, even though they could perfectly well afford a vet, he explained.

'How do you manage to keep so calm?' I asked.

'Ah, that's the value of philosophy. You should try reading Seneca,' he added.

Seneca? I had always thought that was something you took to make you regular.

Still Practising

'Seneca believed that it is by learning not to aggravate the world's obstinacy through our own responses that we achieve wisdom.'

'Right,' I nodded.

'You find most of the philosophers have something to offer in dealing with everyday life. As do most religions. It's the selection that's difficult and the obstinacy of most adherents in refusing to see good in any other belief system but their own.'

There followed the first of many fascinating discussions with Andy, only cut short when Roy returned with two new-born kittens that had survived an attack – probably by a fox, Roy said, looking at the damage.

Roy was a couple of years older than me. Nothing fazed him. He took everything in his stride – gentle on the outside, tough in the middle. He knew the area we covered like the back of his hand. Quiet, and not one to jump to conclusions before he'd thought everything through, he was just the sort of person you want to have on your side in a crisis. I never saw a difficult situation that Roy couldn't handle.

During the hour I was in the night-duty room that first evening hardly five minutes went by without the phone ringing. Not long after Roy returned, news came in of a badly injured dog that would have to be put down. This wasn't the kind of thing Andy liked doing, and he sighed as he pulled on his anorak and said he'd see me tomorrow.

Chapter Eleven

I woke up early, with the dull hum of traffic in my ears; I had left the bedroom window wide open as the night was hot. It was not the sound I was used to – in Canterbury it had been blackbirds.

In the early morning light I wandered around the flat, prince of all I surveyed. The shower was good and strong and the towels were big, if a bit rough. When I had got back from downstairs the night before, all I had wanted to do was to crash out, but first I had to make the bed up; a note by the fridge said that I would find linen in the airing cupboard in the hall. When I pulled back the coverlet to put on the sheets I discovered what I knew was called a duvet but had never actually seen before. Times really were a-changing, as Bob Dylan said.

The sitting room had two settees and one easy chair. The carpet was green, although nothing else was – certainly not the view outside, which was the proverbial concrete jungle. I decided the flat could do with some plants; there was certainly enough light. Everything looked very new, as in fact it was – like the building itself, only three years old. I couldn't get over the size of it and kept wandering around, looking into cupboards and out of the big picture windows, though the view was better sitting down, then you didn't see the wasteland that surrounded the building. In later years the hospital would be at the centre of a brand new estate planted with plane trees, but in the early seventies it was a very unfriendly-looking place indeed.

By eight o'clock I could wait no longer and went down to reception. I was due to meet my new boss, Tony Self, at ten but Trevor Bryant, my old buddy from the Royal Veterinary School had told me he would get in early, and he was true to his word.

'Welcome aboard, Maestro,' he said, giving me a slap on the back. Trevor had been a year below me at college but our paths had crossed when he had been on the entertainment committee and I was involved in security for the various rock concerts the students' union had put on and we had become friends. It was Trevor who had tipped me off about the job at the Harmsworth. Just where the name 'Maestro' came from I never knew.

'Met anyone yet?'

'Roy and Andy last night.'

'Ah yes, and how did you get on with our in-house philosopher? No slacking in the grey cells department there.'

Nor, I should add, was there with Trevor, it was just that he didn't show it, with his open manner. Even his horn-rimmed glasses failed to give him gravitas, but just made him look like a very tall Buddy Holly. He loped across to reception – he was a good 6 foot 3 inches – had a word with the nurse on duty, and then loped back. 'The boss has been held up apparently, and I am to give you the royal tour in his place. He'll be in this afternoon.'

The first stop was the wards, the rooms at the back of the building that housed the different kinds of animals. There were four, plus an isolation ward. First was the cat ward, where two sides of the room were made up of stainless steel cages, nearly all of which were full. Trevor went along them, flipping the cards attached to clips. 'Yellow cards mean the animal has an owner, white means strays, but Mary will go through all that with you later.'

'Mary?'

'Head nurse. Tartar with a heart of gold. Tony Self's shadow. Don't even think of saying anything against him in her presence or you'll be dogfood.'

Then we came to the dog ward, with bigger cages. Their occupants hardly made a noise, except for one awful case – a dog with hardly any hair at all, and scabby and blotched skin showing through over two-thirds of its body. It pawed at the bars and barked and whined demanding attention. I went over and talked to it.

'OK, old feller, what seems to be the matter?'

It was mange of some sort. Yet how had it come to be in such a dreadful condition? It must have been getting that way for several months, and yet this wasn't a stray. There was a yellow card attached to it.

'I know,' Trevor said, raising both his hands in the air. 'He came in yesterday afternoon. It's just unbelievable, but not that uncommon, I'm afraid to say. You'll get used to it.' But I never have. Most of the others were less distressing – broken limbs, post-surgery cases mainly.

The third ward, with a mixture of medium- and larger-sized cages, was used for either dogs or cats. Then it was on to Ward 4, mainly exotics. In veterinary terminology this doesn't mean exotic in the Tarzan sense, but covers anything that isn't a cat or a dog, from budgerigars to snakes, hedgehogs to hamsters. Over half of the cages in Ward 4 that morning had rabbits in them – one of the most common pets in London, certainly.

We by-passed the isolation ward, as that required putting on rubber shoes and we didn't have time. Trevor said that it was comparatively empty – just two cases of cat flu, if nothing had come in over the weekend.

He talked me through the set-up. There were three vets on site with two part-timers, making for a one in five rota – extraordinarily civilized for the times. Operations were done in the morning, consulting was in the afternoon. It was very busy, he explained, with up to 120 consultations in a day, shared by the two consulting vets. I thought he must be exaggerating: in Canterbury a surgery of ten was bad enough. The consulting rooms were set one each side of the dispensary, which would be staffed by a nurse, he explained. A little hatch connected us to them. The rooms themselves were huge, much bigger than I had been used to.

Then it was off to the operating theatres at the rear of the building, away from the noise of reception. There were two of them and a prep room, where the pre-med is given and simple procedures such as blood tests and stitch-ups are carried out. Off that was the X-ray room. All animals in need of an X-ray have to be anaesthetized; unlike with humans, where the procedure is conducted by radiographers, everything was done by a qualified vet.

In the corridor Trevor introduced me to Jim Halliwell, a well-built man in uniform, one of the many RSPCA inspectors, then went off with him to arrange for one of his cases to be admitted. Essentially the job of the inspectors is at the heart of what the RSPCA is all about – to prevent cruelty to animals – though in practice, by the time they're involved it's too late. They're more like policemen than paramedics, which is why they wear uniforms, and if there's one quality that's essential in an inspector, it's a strong nerve – and a strong nose. The conditions that some of these animals are kept in defy belief. A dog driven mad by the cruelty of its owners can be far more dangerous than a criminal. Inspectors weren't attached to any particular hospital or clinic, but they would drop in from time to time, if there was something they needed help with, or something we needed to know about, and naturally we got to know them well. Only a percentage of the calls to the hospital were from owners concerned for the health of their pets; the majority were, and still are, about strays and alleged cruelty – though some were just dogs barking, which we can do nothing about.

The inspectors kept in touch with the hospitals through a radio, run by Securicor, so that we would have some warning if they were bringing an animal in and – if it was at night, which it often was – to alert the vet on call. The vet was needed not just for his skill in the surgery or to pre-scribe drugs, but often to give a statement relating to the alleged cruelty, what's called in legal parlance 'a statement of suffering'.

'German shepherd kept chained up in Stoke Newington,' explained Trevor when he came back. 'Neck is a real mess apparently and head looks as if it's found itself the wrong side of a boot once too often. Jim'll be bringing it in later today, when he's got police back-up to go in. Owner's a known nasty piece of work.' He sighed heavily. 'Right. Up to the centre of all action for a coffee?'

I looked at him quizzically.

'The nurses' common room, Maestro.'

The common room was directly underneath my flat I realized. It looked like a hospital waiting room except for the television at one end, and the mess of magazines and empty coffee cups lying about. Two nurses looked up as we went in. Trevor asked if there was any chance of a coffee, as he wanted to introduce the new vet. We would be back in two ticks, he said.

Still Practising

'Women,' said Trevor. 'Whoever got this idea about them being natural home-makers? Natural mess-makers more like. Excluding Susannah of course, who is the proverbial exception that proves the proverbial rule.' I had not yet met his wife. We went through into the kitchen next door, where a small, round woman with hair as springy as a Brillo pad had her hands deep in a brown bowl of flour.

'Mrs Purser, this is Mr Grant, the new vet on the team.'

'Pleased to meet you I'm sure,' she said.

'Mrs Purser is responsible for giving us a delicious lunch every day, aren't you Mrs P?'

'Don't think you can butter up an old woman with that smooth talk you got off the telly.'

'Mrs P, how can you say that? You know I never watch television.'

Ignoring this last remark she turned to me. 'Anything you don't like, Mr Grant?'

Squid, oysters, snails – I didn't imagine they'd be on the menu. 'Nothing I can think of, thank you Mrs Purser.'

'So what delights have you for us today Mrs P?' Trevor asked.

'Steak and kidney pudding, carrots and boiled potatoes.' Just as I thought.

One room on was the laboratory and next to that was the drugs room. The night staff room I already knew. Then it was back to the nurses' common room for our coffee. At that time there were about sixteen employed at the hospital, all of them except Mary – Tony Self's 'head girl' – younger than me.

When Trevor had to go downstairs to do the morning's operations, I offered to carry on with some routine blood tests that needed to be done. Time flew by; before I knew it, it was time for my first appointment with the boss. I hadn't seen Tony Self since we shook hands the day he offered me the job.

'Sorry I wasn't here this morning, but you know Trevor, I gather, so he doubtless eased you in.'

Tony was one of the old brigade, always immaculately turned out, with a grey suit and white shirt and highly polished shoes into which he put shoe trees when he changed into his operating gown and rubber boots. He had graduated at the end of the war and was now in his late forties. Although Trevor was probably taller, Tony gave the sense of being much bigger. He had a definite presence and was every inch the boss, so there was no tendency to argue, particularly as I soon learned that he had a low flash point and would fly into a rage when things went wrong. It was rarely directed at anyone in particular but usually involved much shouting, and he would get very red in the face. Sometimes I worried that it would lead to a heart attack but it never happened. It was just his way of letting off steam. I soon learned that on a one-to-one basis Tony was as kind a person as you could wish to meet, and always very supportive. He was without doubt one of the best bosses I ever had.

It never ceases to surprise me when doctors – or vets – smoke, and thirty years ago a great many of them did, including my new boss. Even by the early seventies the dangers of smoking were well known, but I suppose that like many non-smokers I underestimate the addictive properties of nicotine. At least Tony knew what he was doing and tried to minimize the noxious effects of tobacco – tar levels in those days were very high – by using a cigarette holder, which with his immaculate turn-out managed to give him a slightly theatrical look. He was very much the David Niven of the veterinary world.

'Now look, David, although I run this place, in essence I'm still a veterinary surgeon, just as you are, and I try never to forget that. Though here at the Harmsworth, you'll find you have as much to do with people as with animals. And you mustn't let it get you down, you'll find yourself faced with situations that are neither pleasant nor within your control. My door is always open, David. Remember that.'

He offered me a cigarette, and I shook my head. 'Very wise,' he said. 'Have you met Mary yet?' I shook my head.

'Heart of gold and nerves of steel, Mary,' he said. 'And take my advice, she's the best resource we've got here at the Harmsworth, as sure as God made little green apples. I know you don't have much experience in our area, so don't worry about asking her questions. That's why I'm putting you two together, at least for a few days. You don't need me to tell you, cats and gerbils present different problems from cows and sheep, and there's no point pretending you know what you're doing when you don't.' I nodded.

'So, welcome over. Any questions? Flat OK? Right, well I won't hold you up. I noticed the queue was stretching round the building when I came in. You better get going.'

I thought he was joking, but when I came down the main stairs into the reception hall I couldn't believe my eyes. There must have been fifty people there. Trevor was already in the next consulting room with a client and gave me a wave and mouthed what looked like 'Have fun.'

Three days earlier I had been on a farm down on the marshes doing a pregnancy diagnosis. Now here I was in inner London facing what looked like central casting for an episode of *Till Death Us Do Part*. The contrast was incredible: from one client the previous Friday, to fifty by the end of my first afternoon at the Harmsworth, although Trevor tried to convince me it was only forty and that he had done more than half the hundred that were seen between us that afternoon. The individual workload in the early seventies at the Harmsworth was far heavier then than it is now, largely because then we had two fewer vets on the team which meant we only held one surgery, which was every weekday afternoon.

Karen, the nurse on duty, handed me a yellow card. Name: Miss Queenie Tuck. Species: Cat, tabby Sex: male Name: Blackie. I dusted off my consultation smile as the door opened. 'Hello, what can I do for you?' I asked.

But no sooner were the words out of my mouth than I sensed something was wrong. As well as a fraying wicker cat basket held together by electric cable, Miss Tuck was carrying three brown paper carrier bags and was wearing slippers. She also had what until then I had only seen Duncan wear in real life, a tamoshanter, although admittedly he only ever wore his in the winter.

Miss Tuck wasn't looking at me at all. She was wandering round the room looking at the walls, looking under the table. The woman was clearly mad. Then the penny dropped. The cheery smile, the mouthed 'Have fun.' Trevor had set me up. My first day, my first consultation, and I'd been set up. I quickly looked down the notes. Miss Tuck was by no means a first-time visitor: the notes ran to two pages. She put the cat on the table.

'How can I help?'

'He wants something.'

'I see. So, what does he want?'

'I don't know.'

The cat sat placidly in the middle of the examination table licking its paws then turning its attention to its bottom. 'So what do you think it is that he wants?'

'I don't know, that's why I brought 'im.'

'What do you think he wants?'

'He keeps asking for something. He wants something and I can't give it to him.'

'Is he eating?'

'Oh yes he's eating.'

'Is he sneezing?'

'No. Not sneezing.'

'Is he coughing?'

'No. He just wants something.'

'What does he want?'

'I don't know, that's why I've brought him.'

I had felt the cat all over, looked at its eyes, its tongue, its teeth. There was nothing wrong with it. I looked at the clock on the wall. Nearly ten minutes had gone. I could feel panic rising like floodwater. At this rate, I thought, I'll be here at midnight. I'd soon learn that just to keep up, I would have to keep consultations down to four minutes each.

Just at that moment I caught sight of Trevor's face at the hatch, the far side of the dispensary that separated the two consultancy rooms. He was looking particularly cheery, I noticed, and appeared to be mouthing, 'The normal.'

The normal? I looked down at the notes again. An injection of vitamin B12.

One minute later and I had a satisfied customer. 'Thank you,' Miss Tuck said, and left. The normal!

Hardly had Miss Tuck closed the door when the nurse handed me another card. Bridey Donovan, it read. The door opened and the first thing I saw was a rear view. She appeared to be pulling something which turned out to be an old-fashioned pram in which were two dogs and three cats. The dogs were attached to the pram by leads, the cats were in baskets.

'Mrs Donovan, how can I help?'

'It's Miss but you can call me Bridey.'

'Right. Well Bridey. Which of these . . . ?' I gestured towards the pram.

'It's Marmeduke,' she said undoing the leather strap on one of the baskets. 'He isn't himself. Not eaten for days now. Doesn't even move.'

Marmeduke was a marmalade cat. I gently lifted him out of the basket. 'You're quite right, Bridey. He's not at all well.'

Marmeduke's eyes were runny and so was his nose. 'Has he been sneezing?'

'A bit.'

Gently holding him by the scruff of the neck I took his temperature. Just as I thought. A fever.

'I'm afraid he's got flu. I'll give him a shot of antibiotic to stop any secondary infection developing, and some antibiotic eye cream.' Although antibiotics won't touch the flu virus, they're useful in preventing infection developing in the sinuses and turning into sinusitis.

'But other than that it's just a question of nursing.'

Bridey smiled broadly. 'Nursing. I'm good at that.'

I wasn't entirely convinced that she knew what I meant by nursing. 'You'll need to keep him warm and try to get him to eat. Flu will have taken away his sense of smell, so he'll need to be tempted with strong-smelling food, like sardines or tinned salmon.' As I was talking I was cleaning up his face with a moistened tissue. 'Do you have any Vick or Vaseline in the house?' Bridey nodded.

'Good, well try rubbing a mixture of that under his nostrils. The vapours should help clear his nasal passages so he'll be able to smell better.' I paused. 'How many cats have you Bridey?'

'Marmeduke, Morris, Mamie, Midge, Errol, Duke and Blossom,' she counted them on her fingers.

'I make that seven.'

'Yes, that's it. Seven.'

'Well, it's best to keep Marmeduke away from the others until he's better. Have they been vaccinated Bridey?'

'Too many.'

'Well, even so, I would strongly advise you to do so.'

She appeared not even to notice I was talking but was delving into a large shopping bag.

'Would you like to hear one of my poems?'

Before I could even get my head round this unusual request, Bridey Donovan picked up Marmeduke and began to recite.

> To survive the winter and to die in spring,
> Oh sparrows what a monstrous thing.

'Well, I don't think you should be too pessimistic about Marmeduke's chances of survival anyway.'

'That's just the first verse. There's more.'

'Perhaps next time Bridey.'

'I'll write out the words, shall I?'

'That would be very kind,' I said as I opened the door and helped push the pram out.

Next was Mrs West with three kittens her daughter had found in a bag by the canal. Someone had tried to drown them but failed. They were all thin and in a pretty poor way, but her daughter was determined to keep them. She was obviously quite well-to-do, but in the circumstances the staff had decided she – or rather the kittens – qualified for RSPCA help.

Next was another cat who wasn't eating. One look at his

teeth told me why. I arranged for him to be admitted to have them all extracted.

Next was a limping dog. I couldn't see any damage, but there was a dark mark on a pink paw. I looked closer. Surely that couldn't be a burn, a cigarette burn. What was I to do? I arranged for a nurse to bandage it up and asked her to keep those notes back.

It was all such a shock: the people, the animals. In Canterbury people may not have been rich, but there wasn't this poverty.

'How many more to go, Karen?' I asked around five o'clock. I had been at it three hours, but it felt more like ten.

'Not many. Another dozen.' Another dozen! I couldn't remember having done a dozen a day in Canterbury. 'You should be through by six. Anyway you're winning. Down to eight minutes this last lot.'

My trouble was that I was by nature a sprinter and, as I was quickly discovering, this required the pacing skills of a marathon runner.

These people didn't have cars, as many of the Canterbury clients had had, and that first afternoon I got used to animals arriving in anything from duffel bags to pushchairs and prams. Then came Mrs Wilkinson.

'Hello Mrs Wilkinson. How can I help you?'

I looked around for an animal but couldn't see one. Mrs Wilkinson, a woman anywhere between 35 and 55, was carrying a vacuum cleaner in an old-fashioned shopping basket on wheels. 'It's Tracy.'

'Tracy?' I repeated.

'I'd slipped out for a quick fag then came back to vacuum the living room then Tracy says where's Elvis? And I says, whatjamean? And she says I left him 'ere. Where is 'e? Well, I says I dunno. But then I remembers sucking up some mess in the corner with the tube. You know, no brush just the tube. Good for corners and doing the grate.' By this time she was holding the vacuum cleaner in her arms like an oversized toddler.

'You mean you think you vacuumed up the gerbil?'

'S'right.'

The body of the cleaner was solid, not like the upright Hoover my Mum used to wield. I put it on the table. 'Do you know how this undoes, Mrs Wilkinson? I mean, when you change the bag? There is a bag, I take it.'

Without saying anything she turned it over and pointed to a sliding mechanism. 'Mind if I have a fag?'

'I'm sorry, this is a no-smoking area.'

Mrs Wilkinson continued jigging from foot to foot.

Once I had managed to prise it open I took out the bag, which was not made of paper, but some sort of loosely woven material. I bent down and listened for any signs of life. No sound. The bag obviously hadn't been emptied for months and by now dust was spilling out everywhere. I asked Karen if she could find an old newspaper, then laid it out, put the bag on it and found a scalpel.

'Just what do you think you're doin'?' Mrs Wilkinson's foghorn voice reminded me of a famous actress called Peggy Mount.

'Opening the bag.'

'You can't do that. Where'm I supposed to get a new one from, eh?'

'Mrs Wilkinson. The entrance to this bag is too narrow for me to get my hand in.'

'The other end. That's where we always empties it.'

Sure enough the other end had a metal clamp across it.

Carefully I eased off the clamp. More dust. Inside everything was felted together. Carefully I prised it away from the bag and it came out more or less in a piece – the size and shape of a cricket bat without the handle. Then, at the end, where the tube would have been, was the inert form of a gerbil. What a way to go, I thought ruefully.

'Elvis!' Mrs Wilkinson screeched. 'Is 'e dead?'

Until that moment I had assumed he was, but at the sound of her voice, the gerbil woke up, and angry at having been disturbed in the nice little nest he had made for himself promptly gave me a hearty nip.

'Well, Maestro,' Trevor said, giving me a playful punch later as I was helping myself to a plaster from the first aid box in the prep room, 'I see you got landed with old Queenie Tuck.'

'As if you didn't know.'

'Quite a character, eh?'

'Oh you mean compared to the others? I must have done about fifty consultations, forty of whom were barking.'

'Rubbish. I did fifty, you did about forty max.'

'Is it always like this?'

'You think I managed to wheel them all in just to give you a hard time on your first day? Dream on. Anyway, you survived.'

'Just.'

'Fancy a beer?' I certainly did. I had just remembered it was my birthday.

Chapter 12

I woke up thinking about the dog with mange I had seen the day before during my tour of the wards. It must have been three months since the symptoms first appeared – I couldn't believe how anyone could have let it get to that state.

Surgery didn't start until nine o'clock and I made my way round the back of the building. A nurse called Janine was already doing the drug rounds while Gill whom I had met when I arrived was giving the dogs their breakfast.

'I know, terrible isn't it?' Janine said as she saw me reading the notes. The dog's name was Biff, and he was just under nine months old. Unfortunately secondary infection had already set in and he was in a really bad way, yelping and clawing at the bars on the cage.

'Has he had a skin scraping yet?' I asked.

'Not yet, no.'

'Well, put it on my list and I'll do it this morning,' I said.

There are two kinds of mange in dogs, demodectic and scarcoptic, both caused by parasitic mites. A major difference is that demodectic mange is caught from the mother at birth, and scarcoptic mange can be caught by any dog from any other, and is highly infectious.

In those days the treatment differed, depending on the kind of mange, and it was important to know which type it was. The symptoms of both are loss of hair and reddening of the skin but scarcoptic mange is much itchier. When a large area of skin is affected, however, it cripples the immune system and because Biff's mange was so far advanced that is just what had happened; as a result his skin was a mass of infected sores which were obviously driving him crazy. When it has gone this far demodectic mange can look like scarcoptic to the naked eye. And although Biff had been put on antibiotics to deal with the infection, the mange itself – the parasite – remained untreated as it would have to wait until a diagnosis was made, which involves scraping some of the skin and examining it. Only under a microscope can the two different kinds of mites be clearly differentiated. Although both have four sets of legs, the demodectic mite is cigar-shaped and the scarcoptic mite is rounder.

An hour later Janine brought Biff in to the prep room, just along the corridor from Ward 2. Ill though he was, he was straining on the lead. We lifted him up on to the table and I took a No. 10 scalpel which I had already covered with liquid paraffin, and scraped it along his skin. When Janine took him back I transferred the material which had stuck to the liquid paraffin to three slides then went up to the laboratory to see what was happening under the micro-scope. Sure enough, there they were, a textbook example of demodectic mites – dozens of them. I went back downstairs to get the treatment started immediately.

In those days the treatment for demodectic mange was extremely laborious and time-consuming. Every day a lotion was applied to one third of the body, the next day it was applied to another third and so on, as it was too toxic to be applied to the whole body at once. And this would go on for three months. Even now it still takes three months to clear, but treatment consists of a bath once a week.

It was only my second day at the Harmsworth but already I felt completely at home. Although we were surrounded by the victims of disease and neglect, there was a wonderful atmosphere among the staff. We were all young and there was always someone to chat to during rare quiet moments, and at the end of the day, without fail, there would be one voice calling out, 'Anyone fancy a drink?' The local pubs, however, were not a patch on the Spotted Cow – nor, come to that, was the beer. The country pubs in Kent retained their locally brewed ales but in London, it seemed, everything was the same.

A few nights after I arrived, I had just finished writing a letter to Caroline and was feeling a bit low. Throughout the evening I had been dimly aware of the phone ringing downstairs, so I decided to look in on Andy and Roy in their lair. I took the fire escape route to the floor below and knocked on the door.

It was opened by an elderly man with a shock of white hair and a beard.

'Oh. I thought Andy . . .' I began.

'You must be the new vet,' he smiled and stretched out his hand.

'Yes. David Grant.'

'Pleased to meet you, David. My name's Bill. Bill Kinnear. I man the phones. Used to go out but not so much now. I let Andy and Roy take the glory.'

The phone rang, and he motioned me to shut the door.

'Harmsworth Memorial Hospital.'

Bill was stocky, and with his white hair and beard a bit of a Father Christmas figure. He must have been a good sixty or more.

'I'm sorry, my dear,' he continued, 'but I don't have the answer to that . . . How long has he been in? . . . Well, my dear, I'm afraid the office is closed at the moment. Might I suggest you call back tomorrow morning after nine?'

He put the phone down. 'Sometime you wonder about people's intelligence,' he said. 'That woman wanted to know how her cat was getting on that came in with a broken leg three days ago. Not exactly life-threatening is it?' He looked at his watch. 'And it's nearly ten o'clock, the time when most honest Christian folk should be abed. Or at least not wasting my time.'

Bill had been with the RSPCA for forty years and was nearing retirement. A few years before he and his 'better half' had moved to Portsmouth and he had to commute three times a week.

'That reminds me; time I gave the missus a tinkle.' I got up to leave. 'No, no. That's all right, David. Stay where you are. Just a word before she goes to bed. A tradition you might say. A quick goodnight sort of thing.'

He pointed to the kettle. 'Care to join me in a cuppa? Perhaps you could put the kettle on while I call her.'

Just as he said, it was only a quick call. I turned my back but of course I could still hear every affectionate word.

'Come next July we'll have been married forty years,' he said when he put the phone down. 'That's something isn't it?'

I had to agree that it was.

Too old for active service in the war, Bill had served as an ARP warden in the London blitz. He had a fund of stories, though that night I just heard the one about animals he had rescued and the horse he had seen killed by lightning.

It was Andy's night off and Roy was out on a call in Hoxton, on the edge of the City. I stayed chatting with Bill until Roy got back.

That night in bed I lay thinking about the difference in our two lives. Bill had spent his childhood in the shadow of the First World War, had lived through the depression of the thirties, and then had a brother and a sister killed in the Second World War. I had been born just as that war had ended and, although my family were only working people, there had never been the terror of poverty that Bill had known. And although there was always talk of a Third World War against the Soviet Union when I was growing up, it never really touched my generation as we had no experience of war, except in films. Bill left school at fifteen. I had had a grammar school education and had gone to university without it costing my parents a penny. And here I was, a fully qualified vet while Bill was just a driver. Yet who was the happiest? Me with my trail of glamorous girlfriends, or Bill with Phyllis, his wife of forty years, four children, six grandchildren and another on the way.

'Ah, David.' Tony Self caught me by the shoulder. I had been at the hospital just over a week and it was not the first time he had stopped and had the occasional word with me – the how-are-you-getting-on sort of chat – but there was something about the way he said my name and the glint in his eye that made me realize that this was different. 'There's a mongrel bitch with stones in her bladder. Thought you might like to have a go. Mary will fill you in.' With that he was gone.

My first operation. I immediately made for the flat. Over the past week or so I had done a few stitch-ups in the prep room, but that was it. Before I found Mary I wanted to get up to speed. Although *Surgery in the Dog and Cat* by a man called Ormrod had been my bedtime reading since I arrived at the Harmsworth, I had not reached bladder stones yet. They are caused by the build-up of minerals, predominantly phosphate, around small foreign bodies in the bladder, much the same phenomenon that comes into play with an oyster, though there the result is the rather more valuable pearl.

At Canterbury each vet usually saw an animal through from diagnosis to treatment. It was rarely like that at the Harmsworth – there were just too many animals. After reading through the appropriate chapter, I went downstairs and sauntered towards the prep room, where I knew I would find Mary. She looked her usual efficient self, not a hair out of place. Although I thought I too looked the picture of composure, Mary obviously thought differently. 'Nothing to worry about, Mr Grant. I'm sure you'll do splendidly.' In all the years I knew her, Mary never called me anything but Mr Grant.

Before the operation itself, I did an X-ray just to confirm the diagnosis, while Mary filled me in on the background to the case.

Cassie's owner was Mr Molloy, who had been planning to travel to Ireland for his father's 92nd birthday when he noticed blood in her urine. He was worried that he would have to cancel because there would be no one to look after her. He loved that dog and there was no way he would leave her.

Mary clipped the x-ray plate up against a light box for us both to see when it was developed. And there were the stones: overlapping circles of solid white clearly visible inside the bladder.

It was some time since I had been involved in the ritual of the operating theatre, and ritual it certainly felt like that day – sacrificial ritual.

Vets wear green operating gowns in the same way as surgeons do, with rubber boots and sterile gloves. The only difference is that on the whole we do not wear masks, as the wound breakdown rate on animals is virtually nil and few veterinary procedures warrant them. Wound breakdown is when the wound does not heal which happens when infection creeps in. Surgeons wear masks to stop their own germs infecting the wound, but as human diseases rarely affect animals, this does not apply with vets.

Cassie was now ready for the operation. I had already given her an anaesthetic before the X-ray – unlike humans, dogs cannot be told to stand still and hold their breath. First I had injected an anaesthetic into a vein and then I had fed a flexible tube down into her wind pipe that delivered the anaesthetic gas that would keep her asleep until the operation was over. It was Mary's job to monitor the anaesthetic.

After the diagnosis had been confirmed, Mary had shaved Cassie's abdomen and now she was lying on her back on the operating table, covered with a sterile drape with a hole in it, through which the operation would be carried out. There was no doubt about the diagnosis: her bladder felt like a bag of marbles.

Then, more calmly than I could have imagined, given I had not done anything like this before, I took a scalpel from the tray Mary had put on top of the surgical table, which had itself been covered by a green cloth. Then I made an incision in Cassie's abdomen, right in the centre along the linea alba, the white line of fibrous tissue where all the muscles of the ventral abdomen meet. An incision here is almost bloodless and it proves a firm anchor for stitches later. First I cut through the skin, then through the muscle. Suddenly there it was, the bladder, looking decidedly wrinkled, irritated by the presence of the stones for what had probably been several months.

I took a breath, then cut into the bladder itself. And there they were, the cause of all that pain, looking like beautiful eggs in a nest. I turned my head towards Mary, who gave me an approving nod.

'Mr Self usually takes them out with these,' she said pointing to what looked like a pair of sugar tongs among the tray of surgical instruments she had laid out for me. Once the stones were out, all that remained was to sew the bladder up, then sew up the muscle and skin along the line of the original incision. And that was it. Mary beamed and I gave a great sigh of relief.

'Well, Mr Grant. That was all right now, wasn't it?' she said. And I hoped the word about Mr Grant would find its way back to Mr Self.

But throughout the afternoon there was a niggle at the back of my mind that I must have done something wrong, and when I got back from the pub later that night, I went in to see how Cassie was doing – to see if she was still breathing. She was; she had even come round sufficiently to roll over on her back and show off her stitches as I gave her ears a scratch. She wasn't well enough to travel to Ireland, however, and, as it turned out, Mr Molloy's father died peacefully a few months later. Cassie never had a recurrence of the problem and died herself at the ripe old age of sixteen. I know because not only did Mr Molloy bring me a bottle of Irish whisky as a thank you, but he sent me a postcard every Christmas from then on, wherever I was.

It is extraordinary what success can do. After Cassie I took to the operating theatre like a duck to water. A major difference between farm-animal and small-animal practice is that when you are out on a farm, whether it is day or night, you are on your own, and that can be very unnerving if you are as inexperienced as I was when I started, especially when you are dealing with animals that are worth an awful lot of money on the one hand and perfectly capable of killing you on the other.

I had always complained to whoever would listen that I had never even learnt how to spay a cat. That was about to be rectified.

The cat in question was a pretty tortoiseshell called Crackers who had had one litter of kittens. Crackers was so pretty that she had had people queuing up to take them. Mrs Hamilton and her would-be cat-owners were extremely disappointed, however, when the kittens turned out to be all male, two ginger and white and two black and white. Tortoiseshell cats are only ever female and Mrs Hamilton did not want to go through the nail-biting business again.

In fact spaying a cat can be surprisingly difficult considering it is such a common procedure. For an experienced vet, however, it rarely causes problems; the key is ensuring that the incision is made in the right place in the flank. The night before I went over and over the illustrations in my new bible until I think I could have drawn them blindfold. Like all veterinary students I had seen a cat spayed, although I had never done one myself – not something that would be allowed to happen these days when qualified vets are proficient from day one.

As instructed, Crackers had been given nothing to eat or drink after six the night before. When she arrived the next morning she was given a pre-med to make her feel dozy, then when we were ready to start, I injected a syringe of anaesthetic into a vein in her leg. Once she was out, the fur on her left flank was clipped by Mary who, once that was done, stretched her out on the operating table and slipped a mask over her nose that delivered the anaesthetic gas. When Mary had finished disinfecting the clipped flank with surgical scrub and spirit, I covered Crackers with a sterile cloth with a hole in it that just left the flank exposed.

I knew that where you make the incision is crucial. If it is done right, then the uterus should just pop right out at you, but if you make the cut in the wrong place, you could miss it as it is only an inch long and the width of a drinking straw. Taking a scalpel off the tray, I cut through the skin, and then down through the muscle, just a small incision, praying that I had judged the position right. Relief. Just as the book had said, the uterus popped right up.

'How am I doing Mary?'

'So far, so good Mr Grant.'

I grinned. Now to find the ovaries. First the left one. That was all right, and I tied a ligature under it. Then the right one. Same thing. Now it was back to the uterus itself. The next thing to do was to clamp arterial forceps across the body of the uterus to stop any bleeding. That done, it can be safely removed. One final ligature and I started breathing again. The final job, after checking that nothing is left behind, is to sew up the muscle, then sew up the skin.

'Okay?'

'Very good.'

Mary was not the only one I had learnt to trust. Right from the beginning at the Harmsworth I knew I was part of a team. If I did not know the answer to a problem, there were always plenty of people to ask, from the other vets to the nurses. Although I was still shattered by the end of every afternoon, it was the humans that were tiring, not the animals.

Bridey Donovan made a second appearance, this time with a dog that had an infected paw, and I met another of the Harmsworth regulars, Mrs Markovich. In spite of her name she was as North London as they come and she had two cats, a male tabby, Butch, and Titch who was black and white – not that I knew that the first time I came across her, as she had only brought Butch.

'It's 'is bum,' she said.

'What's wrong with his – er – bottom?' I said.

''E's always bitin' it, see.'

I had a look. 'I can't see any reason for that – no inflammation,' I said doubtfully.

'Not inflammation, no. I didn't say anyfink about inflammation, no. Just biting. Biting 'is bum. Taint natchral.'

And so it went on. Over the years I was to see Butch again, and it was always ''is bum'. With Titch it was, ''E's gotta froat.' I never discovered anything wrong with either Butch or Titch, 'bum' or 'froat'. In fact they were particularly healthy cats. But she was an old lady who lived on her own. She really only came for the chat.

One hurdle was crossed but another was looming: night duty. It did not help that in Canterbury my first night duty had been a nightmare from start to finish. The evening had started with the death of a dog suffering from gastric torsion; I hadn't known where to start and had had to call in Frank Archer, the senior partner, who had conducted an emergency operation. Although he did everything he could, and the operation was a theoretical success – the tangled stomach having been unravelled – the patient died; his heart just gave out. The night had ended, I remembered, with a tom cat who had been knocked over in the road but when picked up by the police had gone mad and wrecked their car.

A takeaway from an Indian restaurant recommended by Roy provided supper and I settled down in front of the television, waiting for the phone to ring. The first time it was just Bill Kinnear telling me that it was a quiet night. Half an hour later he rang again. Andy was on his way back with a fox that had been run over near St Pancras Station. It was an extraordinary paradox that after three years in the wilds of Kent I had never come across a fox, a symbol of all that is wild and yet here I was, my first night duty in central London, with a fox as one of my patients.

I was waiting downstairs by the time Andy arrived. The fox had travelled back in the van in the kennel usually used for dogs. I had never been close to one before and the stench was almost overpowering. Now it is a smell I can instantly recognize, even in trace amounts, much to the amusement of visitors if they are being shown round; they can smell absolutely nothing. Most people these days have simply never smelt a fox.

Andy was experienced in dealing with foxes and while I opened the door, he grabbed it for me with heavy-duty gloves. She was a young vixen that had been run over. She was a bit dazed with a graze on her head, but otherwise I couldn't find much wrong; in fact she was in beautiful condition.

'Just a dose of concussion then,' said Andy.

'Well, you're the fox expert, what do you think?'

'I'll expect you'll just need to give her a shot of antibiotic and then we'll release her back where we found her tomorrow night – if you want.'

'Good idea,' I replied. I was rapidly learning to lean on the night staff's experience as well as everyone else's. Between them Andy, Roy and Bill had seen it all, though they never tried to give that impression. In terms of accidents and trauma; what those three didn't know wasn't worth knowing.

If this had been Canterbury, a night on call would have

been followed by two more of the same. One of the great incentives for me when I applied for the job at the Harmsworth was the rota which meant just one night in five, although the next night I volunteered to go with Andy to release the fox. It was my first time in the Escort van, but it was not to be my last.

Railway embankments are a haven for foxes in London, one of the few areas in the metropolis that remain undisturbed by humans. If we released her roughly where she was found, Andy explained, she would be able to find her way back to her cubs.

When we got to the street behind St Pancras Station, where she had been picked up, Andy stopped the van. I must admit that at that moment I felt a bit like I imagined a criminal must feel as we waited and watched till the coast was clear – in this case until there was no sign of any traffic. The last thing we wanted was another accident, and we didn't know which side of the road she would run to, or even if this was near her home territory. Without saying a word we opened the door of the cage and quietly let her slip out into the sultry September night. We need not have worried. She sniffed the air and shot down the gap between two warehouses, giving the distinct impression that she was on home ground.

We drove back with the windows wide open to dispel the pungent smell. 'I suppose you get used to it,' I said.

'The smell of fox? No. That's something you never get used to,' Andy replied. 'It's worse than the back streets of Calcutta, take it from me. Second only to ferret in my estimation.'

The route back to the hospital was through Camden. It was around pub closing time and people were spilling out on to the pavements, splitting into couples. I sighed. It would be a long time before I was walking hand in hand with anyone. Andy nodded when I told him what I was thinking and explained the situation between Caroline and me.

'How old are you?'

Twenty-seven, I told him.

He laughed. 'You're young. Young people aren't designed to stay faithful to one another. So don't expect to.'

'Why do you say that?' This wasn't the usual response of the older generation. They always seemed dead keen on being faithful. Mrs Nightingale was a prime example.

'Experience. And Schopenhauer is quite interesting on the subject.'

I had heard the name Schopenhauer, but frankly he could have been a downhill skier or a composer as far as I was concerned.

'So what does he say?' Perhaps philosophy would have some answers after all.

'He believed that we are split into our conscious and our unconscious selves and that although consciously – intel-lectually – you might want to stay faithful, unconsciously you continue to search for someone with whom you can procreate. The intellect only understands the process suf-ficiently to promote reproduction.'

'But this is nothing to do with reproduction,' I said, feeling distinctly panicky at the idea. Anthony and Jackie, Phil and Sue were one thing, but not me. 'I'm not interested in having any children, at least not yet,' I added.

'Your conscious self might not, but your unconscious self decidedly does. That's the whole point. No one, no man that is, who was in their right mind would want to saddle themselves with children. So while a young man is in love, he is, in effect, not in his right mind. It's just self-delusion.

Everything to do with romantic love is self-delusion. According to Schopenhauer that is.'

But not, I was sure, according to Mrs Nightingale.

But Andy had set me thinking. I had written Caroline two letters, but hadn't heard anything from her. How long did the post take from Toulouse? Had she even arrived safely? I could have called her parents, but . . .

Also, surrounded by so many young females among the staff, it was hard not to look at them as, well, attractive young females. There was one who had a very cheeky grin, but I did not even know her name. I could easily have found out from Trevor, but I knew that if I did that it would be just the first step on a slippery slope. No, I would just have to prove Herr Schopenhauer wrong.

Chapter Thirteen

For the first few days at the Harmsworth it was all I could do to crawl upstairs and crash out in front of the television. But after a couple of weeks, once the novelty of finishing work at a civilized hour began to wear off, I began to think sensibly about doing all the things I had planned to do in my spare time when I first took the job. For a start I realized I was incredibly unfit and would only get worse, as I was no longer walking several miles a day – which is what I must have been doing in Kent if you added it all up, not to mention the sheer physical energy expended when dealing with cows. So one of the first things I did was to get in touch with my old athletics friends from university and one night a week went to Crystal Palace to train.

I was also determined to learn more about classical music. Records are one thing, but now that I was in London I had some of the best classical music in the world right on my doorstep. With just a bit of effort I could experience the real thing. A new weekly magazine was being published called *Time Out*, which gave details of concerts, films, plays, everything you could think of that was going on in London. Written and owned by people my age, it was honest and forthright – if something wasn't any good, they would say so. *Time Out* is still going strong, of course, but now it's a glossy publication; in the early seventies it was no more than twenty pages of roughly printed paper. But just reading it was enough to remind me that there was a whole world out there which had nothing to do with veterinary medicine.

Then there was that other ambition of mine, to learn Spanish. I was sure there was some kind of evening class I could get on in London. After making enquiries at the library, I discovered that the beginner's Spanish class run by the local technical college had already started; the next one wasn't till the new year, the librarian told me, but she gave me the number of a language school in Oxford Street where she thought I might be lucky. And indeed I was.

My teacher, who was called Graciella, was from Argentina, from a town called Mendoza. To call her beautiful is not to get near what she looked like. She was exotic, with lustrous dark hair, smouldering eyes and skin the colour of milky coffee, the sort of looks you couldn't help staring at. But far more important was that she was a very good teacher. It turned out I knew more than I thought I did. All it needed was practice, she said, and I soon found I could say real things – putting together words and ideas to make the beginnings of conversations.

South American Spanish sounds very different from the Spanish spoken in Spain, but as all my experience up to that time had been from the *Daily Express* handbook, this presented no problems at all. In fact quite the reverse: it was probably easier as I had nothing to unlearn and I rapidly got used to Graciella's almost Italian way of speaking: soft, musical and slower than the guttural, lisping, staccato Spanish from Madrid or Torremelinos.

Without realizing it, I was enjoying life to the full again. I was revelling in my work at the Harmsworth: being young and full of energy, I had soon come to grips with the heavy caseload. And, as for the Spanish, it was just as Graciella had said to me, when I spoke to her before the first lesson:

'Learning by a book, Señor Grant, is not the same thing at all as hearing the voice of the language, its nuances of tone and inflection. Never forget the language is about sound and music, not marks on a piece paper. You must let it flow over you, into every part of your body, until it becomes part of you.'

Language is all about culture and because Graciella was Argentinian, she would talk to the class about what she knew, about her home country and the other Spanish-speaking countries of South America. Music and food seemed to be the two things that we ended up discussing. Later we would turn to Latin America's literary heritage, but for beginners it was the perfect introduction. Every week she would bring in one or two records and her portable record player; first we would listen to them just as a musical experience, then we would try to hear individual words in the songs – one or two would always stand out – and finally, with Graciella's help, we would try and make sense of the emotion, the story that the words and music together were trying to convey.

It's not a tradition that is familiar to English ears and the word and stories themselves were often surprisingly harsh. Even dance music like the tango usually had words and most of them told very complicated stories about love and being abandoned. We learned how the tango had emerged from two quite different dances, the Creole waltz that had its origins in Eastern Europe and the Milonga, which was a peasant dance of the pampas. Later I grew to love another South American dance, the cueca from Chile, with its fantastic rhythm. I quickly became fascinated by Latin America and I was determined to do more than just talk about it.

Sometimes fate deals you a karate chop, at other times it's waiting in the wings with a piece of chocolate cake. And one evening as I was walking back to the tube from the Soho café where we all went after the class was over, I was stopped in my tracks by a voice from the other side of the road. 'Granty!'

Only one person called me that. I turned and there, sure enough, there crossing the road was none other than Henry Garcia.

Henry had been a year below me at college, the same year as Trevor in fact, and I hadn't seen him since then. 'Granty, you old reprobate,' he said grasping me in a bear hug. 'Where have you been?'

I told him I was just on my way back from a Spanish class. Of course what he had meant was, where had I been for the last three years. But it was what psychiatrists I think call 'free association'. Although Henry Garcia sounded as English as I did – and in many ways appeared more English than the English – he was in fact Colombian and his real name was Enrique, but everyone, including his Colombian friends, called him Henry. His father had worked for the BBC World Service for years, broadcasting to South America.

Henry told me he was on his way to a Spanish bar at the far end of the Portobello Road where he was going to meet one of his brothers and some Spanish friends. Didn't I know that North Kensington was the Spanish/Portuguese/South American heart of London, with more supermarkets, bars and restaurants than fleas on a dog? I had to admit I didn't.

'Well, no time like the present,' he said. 'The Galicia is the most authentic Spanish bar in London. My car's round the corner.'

As I was soon to learn, the Colombian tradition of hospitality is formidable and there was no way I was getting that tube back to Finsbury Park. Minutes later we were halfway there. I hadn't driven this fast, I realized, since driving with Nick back from the coast to Canterbury in the summer. What was it about vets and cars, I wondered? In less than five minutes we were in the Bar Galicia, at the wrong end of the Portobello Road, under the shadow of high-rise tower blocks.

I knew from the moment I walked in that this was the real thing. It was just like being in Spain. Not only did it look like it, it smelled like it, a mixture of garlic, wine and Spanish cigarettes that is unlike anything else. And the whole evening I never heard one word of English.

As we went in there was much hugging and kissing, and glasses were lined up on the counter top and filled to overflowing. Slices of mountain ham were cut and there were bowls of crisply fried whitebait, eaten in handfuls like crisps, all washed down with sherry, red wine or the only beer on offer – *cerveza*, San Miguel. I noticed that there were no women at all.

Although I understood only about one word in twenty, I had no feeling of being left out and I just let the language wash over me as Graciella had advised, and enjoyed the bottles of cold *cerveza*. Although I never drank anything other than bitter in English pubs, this place didn't feel like England. It felt like being in Spain, and when in Spain . . .

Eleven o'clock came and went and it was gone midnight before Henry suggested it was time to go. 'My wife will be wondering where I am,' he explained. Wife! Not only did I discover that Henry was married, but also that he had a baby son. I couldn't believe it: Henry the family man.

I should come around and meet them, he said, his voice full of pride. It turned out he lived only a few miles from the Harmsworth. I wondered how he coped: unlike me he was still a student, still at the Royal Veterinary College doing a

PhD. 'But what do you do for money?' I asked.

'I get a small bursary, and Berta works – translation is quite well paid and she can do it from home. But it's not easy that's for sure.'

As we talked, another part of my brain was working overtime. The RSPCA believed in doing everything by the book, and whenever we were a vet down, either through illness or someone going on a course or holidays there was no question of the rest of us just somehow filling in; Tony Self would always get in a locum. It was never for more than a day here or there, but it would help, I reckoned. Henry was a qualified vet and he lived locally. There seemed no reason why he couldn't be one of the names on the list, unless there was a system that I didn't know about. But I thought it better not to say anything until I had had a word with the boss. No point in raising false hopes.

The next day I mentioned Henry to Tony Self. 'Colombian, you say.'

'Yes. But you'd never know it. He's been here since he was four.'

'So English OK then?'

'Totally.'

'Get him to give me a ring and we'll take it from there.'

I waited till afternoon surgery was over, then dashed upstairs to the flat and picked up the phone.

'*Señor Garcia se encuentra?*'

'*Si. Momento, por favor.*'

I nearly dropped the phone. I had spoken Spanish and she had understood!

'*Hola!*'

'*Hola* yourself,' I replied.

'My God, Granty, it's you. This is very impressive. Berta said she didn't know who it was, but didn't suggest it

David Grant

was a Brit, let alone a Brit who until he visited the Bar Galicia was incapable of speaking a word of Spanish. You've got a way to go yet, but I think there's hope.'

'There's certainly hope for you, Henry.'

'Meaning?'

And I told him about the possibility of locum work at the Harmsworth and that Tony Self was expecting his call.

They say what goes around comes around and soon Henry was picking up enough days at the Harmsworth to make a real difference financially, and to gain him valuable experience. At the same time, Berta decided that to say thank you she would always talk to me in Spanish and she insisted that I went round there to keep her company while Henry was upstairs working on his thesis.

Everything about her was tiny, like a bird. And so I called her Bertica, literally 'Little Berta'. She was a lovely person, very well educated and with beautiful manners and, even though my Spanish must have been pretty dire in those early days, she was very long-suffering and never allowed me to speak English with her. We became lifelong friends.

I have always enjoyed the company of women, but being determined to disprove Schopenhauer I had made no attempts to seek out any feminine company. Caroline had eventually written to me and I still wrote to her, but I found it hard to convey the excitement I felt, both at the Harmsworth and in the New World, where I had suddenly stopped being a Little Englander.

Caroline's first letter hadn't arrived till she had been in Toulouse nearly a month. Although I wrote to her regularly, she rarely seemed to find the time and her letters were getting shorter. She talked of things that meant nothing to me – gossip about people she had written about in an earlier letter. I woke up one day in a real state. I had had a dream where we were walking somewhere and I had tried to hold her hand, and she pulled away and said, no, someone might see.

But with Berta and her little boy Alejandro I had the best of both worlds: a generous and kind woman to talk to and laugh with, but completely free of any other emotions. She was a wonderful mother, in sharp contrast to a case that came in towards the end of November.

A call had come through from a little girl called Tracy. It seemed that she was at home alone with her brother and the family cat had crawled in obviously badly injured. The nurse sent out to bring the animal in was Helen, who was only twenty but already fully qualified and fairly experienced. She was often sent out to collect injured animals when the owners couldn't bring them in themselves. The name of the cat was Tammy – in fact she was little more than a kitten, only a year old and great friends with the family's other pet, a mongrel puppy called Spot, who was about the same age.

The two children had been on their own in the house when it had happened. Adam was seven but it was eight-year old Tracy who had had the presence of mind to call the Harmsworth. She had remembered the telephone number was written on an appointment card they had been given at the hospital a few months before, when they had brought Tammy in because she had been rolling about and making strange noises, and, they thought, dying in agony. In fact she was just in season. This is standard behaviour, but it was the first time it had happened. When I looked up the record later I noticed that it was Tony Self who had seen Tammy and advised them that she should be spayed. An appointment had been made (this was the card Tracy had found) but they had failed to turn up.

It was not that unusual to see the nursing staff getting

angry at the way people treated animals, but when Helen returned she was angrier than I had ever seen her. 'Even walking up the garden path, you knew something was wrong,' she said. 'All the other gardens were looked after in some way. But this one, well it looked like –' and she gesticulated out of the window at the desolation that surrounded us at the Harmsworth. 'The garden was filled with broken bits of metal, old planks of wood and weeds as high as my waist – not to mention enough empty bottles to open a pub. And then those two little mites. The boy had to stand on a box to reach the latch. "Where's your Mum?" I said. And they said they weren't sure, but she'd probably be back soon. Oh yes. Like she had been the day before and the day before that, no doubt.'

After examining the cat, Helen had reckoned it was a broken pelvis. And she was right. When I finally got to see her Tammy was in a bad way. She was used to being outside, the children had told Helen. She had been hit by a car but had somehow managed to make her way back to the house. Although they had been told not to open the front door, when they heard her piteous mewing they did. The cat had literally crawled in and was being licked by Spot.

Helen hadn't known what to do. Mike, the ambulance driver who'd driven her to the house, could take the kitten back to the hospital, but what about the children? She had been in the kitchen to wash her hands and it was disgusting, she said. No food, nothing. Just as Mike came back with the cage for Tammy, they both heard a shout, and the parents had returned. Helen said that as soon as they heard the father's voice, the children both cowered behind her.

'Even I was frightened,' she said. 'Both of them were obviously the worse for drink. The mother did nothing much, just stood there swaying. But he was the belligerent kind of drunk, red-faced and swearing and shouting, "What do you think you're doing" though using much stronger language.'

As if in answer, Helen said, there came the unmistakable sound of the little mongrel puppy peeing. At which the father picked it up roughly by the scruff of its neck, opened the door and flung it outside.

'Don't, Tel,' the woman had whined, 'you'll hurt the little bugger.'

'Hurt him? I'll bloody kill him if he messes in our house.'

Just then Helen heard a loud squealing of brakes and a dull thud followed by a high-pitched yelping. 'I just felt sick,' she told me. 'I just knew it was that little dog. He was only a puppy and would have had no road sense. Of course you can imagine what the man did – started blaming the kids. Mike saw everything.'

Spot had a bad fracture in one leg. He could just stand, but the back leg seemed to be swinging free. He was clearly in shock, with blood streaming down his face. Mike and Helen took both animals and left with the sound of the man's voice ringing in their ears shouting abuse, though whether at them or the children, Helen said, she couldn't hear.

Meanwhile, back at the hospital Trevor and I were waiting, having been alerted by Mike over the radio that not one but two injured animals were now on their way in. But then they hit the rush hour. The house wasn't that far away but the Harmsworth is right in the middle of a horrendous one-way system and it was the best part of an hour before they were in Finsbury Park.

As soon as they arrived we were into a set routine that we had done so many times it was like clockwork. With a nurse each we checked each animal over and put them on drips for shock. Then came an injection of pain-killer, and within an hour, as by then they were both stabilized, they were X-rayed.

As Helen had suspected, Tammy had a fractured pelvis which would heal with rest, although she would need to stay with us for at least a week. Fractured pelvis was something I was seeing on a daily basis and always in cats; it seemed to be much rarer in dogs. These patients needed intensive nursing. Often they needed their bladders expressed daily because there was damage to the nerves controlling them. This could go on for ten days or more. Pain-killing injections would be needed every day and the cat would have to be tempted to eat. None of this would be appreciated in any way whatsoever by these particular owners. As I marked up Tammy's notes, I thought of Miss Heskins. I was beginning to miss Miss Heskins – it was a different world.

Meanwhile Spot had fared little better. He had broken the bottom of his thigh bone. This, I was soon to find out, was a very common injury in dogs less than a year old after being hit by cars.

Trevor and I surveyed the X-rays together. 'Bags I put a pin in that tomorrow,' he said.

Trevor was already into double figures with this type of break. He kept a log of all the operations he had done and was often to be seen checking the clinical cards to see how they had got on.

The phone went in the prep room. One of the nurses answered it. 'Trevor, it's for you. Your wife. She wants to know what time you're likely to be home.'

I looked at the clock – it was already eight o'clock. I could hardly believe it was so late. 'A bit of your usual bad timing there, Trev. I was going to offer to buy you a pint.'

'Tell Susannah I'll be back by – er – nine. Tell her I've just got one more thing to do.'

He grinned as we nipped over to our local. With the saloon bar bigger than the Harmsworth's reception area, and a staff never less than five, it was about as far removed from the Spotted Cow as could be imagined. The floor was littered with cigarette butts and music blared from the juke box. In a back room there were four pool tables. Theo's bar skittles and his hard-core dominoes team wouldn't have survived long in this place, I thought. Nor would Theo. But after the day we'd just been through, it would just have to do.

At least the animals were safe now, I thought, as I returned to the flat an hour or so later. I just hoped they wouldn't be abandoned by their owners. Or perhaps, I considered ruefully, that might be the best thing. Then I thought about the children. It would break their hearts. We would just have to see.

Suddenly I was whacked. If truth be told I was still hung over from the party I had gone to with Henry the day before. In England, if you're invited for Sunday lunch then you leave by four. If you're invited for drinks at six, then by 8.30 you should be gone. English parties, whatever kind they are, have a clear beginning and a clear end. Colombian parties, I had just learned, operated to a quite different rhythm.

As I had been invited to lunch I had arrived at Henry's parents' house at about one. However, the food didn't arrive till nearly four, and it was gone midnight by the time I left. Most of the forty or so guests seemed to be family, though it was hard to tell how closely people were related. 'Meet my cousin' seemed a useful way of introducing someone,

one that I sensed was not strictly accurate in the English sense.

That first night when Henry had taken me to the Bar Galicia to meet his brother I had understood about one word in twenty. Now thanks to Berta, it was more like eight words in twenty, which was enough to let me just listen and try to understand, and to forget English altogether.

Not everyone was a relative. Berta had lined up one of her old friends from school in Colombia who had recently arrived in London. Her name was Gloria and she had a degree in psychology.

'Feast' would have been a better name than lunch for the meal we had that day. There was a huge bowl of rice, fish and chicken, like a paella but hotter than any paella I had had in Spain. Then there were dishes of lentils and spicy sausages, and dishes of beans with spicy sausages and dishes of what I later discovered were a vegetable called okra, ladies' fingers, which I didn't like much. Best of all was a whole lamb called *asado criollo*, which had been roasted over a slow ash fire, a bit like a barbecue.

To drink we started with something that tasted a bit like ouzo which was drunk neat. And to follow there was wine and cava, Spanish champagne.

Immediately after lunch, the dancing began. It was quite a surprise; not only the young people were dancing, but everybody, from 5-year olds to grannies – except me that is. The music was salsa – all the rage now, but in 1971 hardly ever heard outside South America. Of course we had talked about salsa in Graciella's class, we had even listened to the music. But I had never danced to it. That was about to change. When Berta came up and took my hands, I shook my head and told her I wasn't really very good at dancing and I would just prefer to watch.

Still Practising

It was the first time I ever saw her roar with laughter – she was usually so polite and restrained. She just pulled me onto the floor and that was it.

In South America, dancing isn't about 'getting off' with someone of the opposite sex. It's simply about the joy of dancing. Although it looked as though there was a lot of flirting going on, it was just part of the dance, not something that led to something else. As soon as the music stopped, the flirting stopped too. The intimacy of the dance was over. You changed partners and the whole thing started again.

Much as I was enjoying myself, I wasn't really very good, and Berta's friend Gloria announced that she would become my dance tutor. Later she announced that she would become my Spanish tutor too. Although Gloria spoke very good English, because Berta had introduced us in Spanish that was the language we continued to use. And in the thirty years we have been friends, we have never had a conversation in English. So began another lifelong friendship. Friendship it started as, and friendship it remained. I'm not really sure why, but somehow romance never entered into it.

Gloria was different from the other Colombian women I was to meet over the years. While the adjectives to describe them would be 'sultry', 'exotic' and 'tempestuous', the adjective that best described Gloria was 'elegant'. She didn't even look particularly South American. She was always elegantly dressed, never flamboyant, as so many South American women can be. In all the years I have known her, for example, I have never seen her in jeans and a jumper.

Now, nearly twenty-four hours later I was still whacked, and just as I was going to bed I remembered the letter from Caroline I had in my pocket. Usually the words 'letter from France for you, David' from the reception staff lifted my spirits. But that morning I had suddenly had a dreadful, sinking feeling. I had looked at the envelope: it was just like all the rest, and yet I decided not to open it and just put it in my pocket. It was the first time I had ever done that.

Now I opened it – just one page, two sides. French paper covered in squares, like the arithmetic books we used to have at primary school, only bigger sheets. The phrases still come back to me after all these years.

'Dear David
This is the letter I thought I would never write. I have fallen in love. He's called Jean-Marie and he's a lecturer here. Not a dirty old man, David, though I know that's what you'll be thinking. In fact he's twenty-eight, only a year older than you, and I think you would like him. In fact when I first met him, I think I was drawn to him because he reminded me of you, though you probably won't thank me for saying so.

I wanted to write to you because you had to know before Christmas. And I just hope that this won't leave you with a gaping hole. Because in fact I won't be coming back for Christmas to Canterbury. As you can imagine, Mum and Dad aren't best pleased either. I'll be spending Christmas with Jean-Marie and his family in the Pyrenees, where they have a house.

So, there we are. I'm really sorry David and we really did have good times, didn't we? I will never forget the animals. Look after yourself.'

I sat numb and angry. Jean-Marie – what kind of a stupid name was that? And even if he was only twenty-eight, how dare this man misuse his power and authority to seduce young foreign students who were so impressionable? I looked up at Janet Potter's painting of the bridge and remembered that day in the summer when we had followed the stream up till we found the place. And how cool it had felt. And how we'd taken our shoes off and dangled our feet in the water.

Bloody Schopenhauer. Caroline's other letters were stacked up behind the toaster in the kitchen. I got them, added this latest one and put them in the wardrobe, under a pair of waders that I was never likely to use. It didn't do to be sentimental, I decided. At least I now knew the name of the nurse, the one with the smile. Terri, she was called.

I went downstairs and knocked loudly at the drivers' door. 'It's open,' Andy said. Well, that was one good thing. I hadn't been down to the night-duty room for days and I hadn't a clue who would be on duty. 'Bloody Schopenhauer,' I said.

'I think you had better sit down.'

Chapter Fourteen

'I'm afraid you won't get much sympathy from Schopenhauer,' Andy told me after giving me a cup of sweet tea – his idea of emotional first aid. When I saw him putting in the sugar I had tried to stop him. 'I don't take sugar,' I said.

'You do tonight,' he told me. 'Sugar is the best treatment for shock.'

'Not philosophy?'

'Well, not Schopenhauer anyway. I might have given you the wrong impression the other night. He was one of the world's great pessimists. He believed that human existence must be a kind of error and that if things are bad today they can only get worse.'

'I don't need to hear that.'

'Like I said.'

'So what should I do?'

'What do you mean?'

'What should I do about it?'

'What do you want to do?'

'I don't know. That's why I'm asking you.'

'You sound like Queenie Tuck, David.'

All the tension of the past half-hour erupted and I laughed as I remembered how my very first patient at the Harmsworth had used the very same words. I laughed and laughed, till tears welled up in my eyes. Sometimes when that happens they can turn into real tears. And if I had been on my own perhaps they would have done.

'I take it you've come across her then,' Andy said when my laughter died down.

'I take it you've come across her then,' I repeated.

'Yes, well. The Harmsworth wouldn't be complete without Queenie. Her presence provides a constant reminder to us all as to the existential nature of life. If she didn't exist we would have to invent her. Everyone needs a Queenie Tuck in their life.'

'Not every week they don't.'

Now it was Andy's turn to laugh. 'Does she really turn up that often?' he asked.

'Probably not. It just feels like it.'

'Life is not about being happy you know, and the sooner you realize that, the happier you will be. If that doesn't sound like too much of a paradox.'

'Who said that? Not Schopenhauer?'

Andy nodded. 'He believed that from the deluded hope of a vague happiness that somehow we all believe we are entitled to, all we get is dissatisfaction. Epicurus believed that happiness is the absence of unhappiness.'

'So how do I get rid of my unhappiness?'

'Pretty basic stuff. By what my granny would call "counting your blessings", David. And you could perhaps take comfort from the fact that having a girlfriend wasn't among Epicurus's list of essentials for a happy life. The most important of these was friendship.'

'But Caroline was my friend. My best friend.'

'Are you sure?'

I sighed.

'David, I've seen you leave here every night for a trip to the pub surrounded by young women. I don't even know all their names – Karen, Janine, Terri, Helen, Gill. And of course there's your old mate Trevor. And Henry, another old mate, and all those other South Americans you've been telling me about. And I don't imagine you flog off to Crystal Palace, race round the track or whatever you do without talking to anyone. Then there is health. Look at you. If you were a dog they'd be entering you for Crufts.

'Epicurus also rated freedom pretty highly. You're young, you obviously love your job, which is comparatively well paid. By any contemporary rule of thumb you are free. You have no major commitments and, even if the unthinkable were to happen and Tony Self gave you the boot, your qualifications would see you right. Finally Epicurus believed that thought was essential for happiness. He was a great believer in thinking things through; even talking about a problem is helpful, and it seems to me that you're quite good at that.'

'But I feel I've made such a mess of this. And Caroline is not the first.'

'Then take a leaf out of Epicurus's book. Don't just dismiss it, analyse what went wrong. And when you say Caroline is not the first, well, from what you told me there may have been other women in your life, but I suspect that up until now you've done the dumping. This is probably the first time you've been dumped. Am I right? You probably won't like hearing this David, but I imagine what you're feeling at the moment is more hurt pride than anything else.'

Andy was right about the hurt pride, but it wasn't strictly true that I'd always done the dumping. Sally had ended our relationship, and so had Angie, though I had to admit they had had enough provocation. What I did know was that I had never felt like this before, as if someone had punched me in the stomach, then made me drink salt water.

A couple of days later I was surprised to see two children in

Still Practising

Ward 3. This was unusual: we didn't encourage visits because there were just too many people and animals involved. It was only when I saw that Helen was with them that I realized who they were. 'So which one is yours?' I asked kneeling down beside the little girl.'

'Tammy.' She pointed at the cat. 'Spot is Adam's though you don't really own animals, do you?' she added.

'No, that's quite true. Though you do have to look after them and it'll be your job to make sure Tammy and Spot get looked after when they get home.'

She nodded solemnly.

'Well, Tammy is doing fine. And all thanks to you being so quick calling the RSPCA. I did the operation on her you know. My name's David.'

'Oh.'

'And a friend of mine, called Trevor, he did the operation on Spot.'

In fact Trevor had done a lovely repair job on Spot's leg. The post operative X-ray showed the pin neatly in place and you could hardly tell where the original break was. My competitive streak, lying dormant now that I was not competing on the athletics track, was fired up. I wanted to be able to repair a fracture as well as that. Thus started a friendly, almost unstated, rivalry which, looking back, was to spur both of us on to the best we were capable of. I suspect Tony watched us with wry amusement, although he was getting the bug too, spurred on by our enthusiasm.

With so many trauma cases coming in it was almost inevitable that a vet working at the Harmsworth would become interested in fracture fixation. I had approached my first few cases with trepidation – with good reason. No other cases expose your fallibility more obviously than the repair of broken bones. If it goes well, then all the world can see your success – a pet running around on four legs without a care in the world. The converse was also unfortunately true. If the case goes wrong the animal might never use that leg again, or at best will need further surgery.

Part of the equation was the owners. If they worked at it, did what they were asked, kept appointments, rested the patient, the omens were usually good. Often, though, none of this happened and in extreme cases the animal simply got run over again.

The two thin, pale, brow-beaten kids turned out to be devoted owners. Every day before and after school they would arrive at the hospital begging to see their pets. In the end the busy nurses took pity on them and let them stay for half an hour or so and hand-feed them. It was good therapy for both the children and their pets, and after a few days I saw a smile for the first time on both their faces. I caught the boy nibbling on some chicken which had been specially cooked for Tammy, who was the slowest to start improving. This careful nursing continued for two weeks, by which time both pets were fit for discharge. They had both put on a lot of weight – which is more than could be said for the kids, who still looked as thin as ever.

There was no way the parents could be persuaded to come and pick up their animals, so in the end Helen volunteered to take them home, taking with her a sack of food paid for by the nurses – enough to feed Tammy and Spot for at least two weeks until the next check up. Helen felt sure – and from what I saw of them I agreed – that the children would see that their pets got all the treatment and rest they needed, so the outlook was good. What did worry Helen was the children themselves – they seemed so neglected, she confided when she came back from delivering the animals back home. 'I just knew the parents wouldn't be there, which was why I asked Magda to take me when I knew the kids would be back from school. And I was right. Magda said she sees it all the time. At least, she said, they didn't have any broken bones themselves. She says she's even called the NSPCC before now.'

Magda was one of the most cheerful people I think I have ever met. She was tiny, not much more than about 5 feet, with dark, curly hair. By the time I met her, I suppose she must have been in her early forties, and pure cockney you would have thought on hearing her talk, but in fact she was Polish. She had come over in 1939, just before the Nazis occupied Warsaw, brought out by an old aunt, her father's sister. The rest of her family were transported and died in Birkenau concentration camp. The aunt had relatives in Whitechapel, in London's East End. No sooner had she arrived in London than the house they were living in was bombed and Magda was sent to Norfolk as an evacuee, but she ran away back to London and somehow found her aunt again. Much to the authorities' dismay, Magda and her aunt stayed in the East End throughout the war, helping Jewish refugees.

Her old aunt had died, aged seventy-five, on the day of the Queen's Coronation, Magda told me with some pride, but not before she had taught Magda to drive. In fact, during the last year of the war, when Magda was only fifteen, she was driving her old aunt about in the car the charity she worked with provided, because the old lady's cataracts meant she could hardly see. If they had known she couldn't drive, she would have been retired, Magda said. Although she had never taken a driving test, she was one of the best drivers I have ever driven with. She could find her way around the labyrinth of streets from Tottenham to Blackfriars, and take a corner like Paddy Hopkirk.

David Grant

Magda's first job had been as a kennel maid at a greyhound track in Wimbledon. But it was south of the river, out of her 'manor' and the dogs came and went. What she wanted was greater involvement with animals. She joined the RSPCA in 1955 and moved to the Harmsworth when it opened in 1967.

Her job had several aspects to it. Like all ambulance drivers she was involved in collecting stray cats and dogs which had been injured in road accidents, and the wildlife she also picked up was quite staggering, considering her patch was central London. There were foxes, ducks, pigeons, starlings, frogs, toads and more hedgehogs than she could remember. The reputation of the RSPCA is such that whenever a member of the public finds an injured animal or bird, they rarely phone anyone else. If the call came into the Harmsworth, Magda would be on her way within minutes.

All ambulance drivers did this, but Magda had another role, one that she had made her own. This involved what were known as 'van treatments', and in the main were for elderly, infirm or bedridden owners who couldn't get the animals in on their own. Magda would go to the house or flat, talk to the old person and get as much of the history as she could, then bring the animal back to the hospital for treatment. She also gave us vets an idea of what conditions were like in the home, whether the owner was up to administering a long-term drug treatment, and so on.

Over the three years she had been at the Harmsworth, Magda had built up a substantial list of old folk who depended on her for just about everything, because Magda loved old people as much as she loved animals. I suppose it was because they were equally vulnerable – but it might also have been because of the debt she felt she owed her aunt.

She had an encyclopaedic memory for streets, and if she

wasn't on an emergency call and found herself in the vicinity of some old person, she would drop in and find out how they were doing and even do essential shopping for them. Cups of tea were her stock in trade, combined with a chat, which was often what they needed more than anything. In the sixties and early seventies, whole communities were being uprooted to so-called new towns, 'London overspill', they called them, places like Basildon in Essex, Basingstoke in Hampshire and Milton Keynes in Buckinghamshire. While young families were happy to go, the older people were not and often had elected to stay where they still had memories, near the graves of their loved ones. The result was a lot of lonely old people.

The numerous broken bones in cats and dogs that were flooding through the doors each day certainly presented a challenge. I felt angry at the sheer neglect of some of them. It was not at all unusual to see the owners walking out of the hospital, taking a dog home after some complicated procedure without even bothering with a lead. No wonder they got run over.

Trevor was really into the orthopaedics and would always bag the fracture cases that came in. I began to wonder how I could catch up. Flicking through the *Veterinary Record* one Friday morning, I saw an advertisement for an orthopaedics course in Davos, Switzerland. It was entitled 'Internal repair of fractures using compression fixation'. Davos sounded exotic – maybe I could learn to ski at the same time. I would need to brush up my O Level German I decided, as I filled in the form to get details of the course.

Two days later Magda came in with a budgerigar with a growth on its wing, which belonged to an old lady in Limehouse. 'Name's Beaky,' she told me. 'Fink you can do anyfing for 'im, darlin'?'

Beaky was about six years old, I reckoned – getting on for a budgie, eight is quite old – and had developed a growth on his wing. The problem was that he wouldn't leave it alone and kept pecking it and making it bleed.

Although she 'wouldn't give you the steam off her tea', Magda said, Flo would cut off her arm if she thought it would save Beaky. Flo was eighty-three and had told Magda that if Beaky died so would she.

Cancers in budgies are quite common and one of the few things I remembered from Frostie's lectures at college were that two-thirds of budgies die of some form of cancer – why, I did not know, not then, not now.

Magda was a battler and, even though I didn't know her well then, I could already sense that she wouldn't take no for an answer.

'I'm not really a budgie expert, Magda,' I explained.

'What? And you call y'self a vet? And don't tell me you fancy having the death of a little old lady on your conscience, eh darlin'?'

The curse of Duncan lives on, I thought.

The problem that first presented itself in relation to operating on Beaky was not the operation itself, but the anaesthetic. While other animals usually had anaesthetic gas pumped down into their lungs via a rubber tube, this was clearly not possible with a budgerigar, however small the tube.

Trevor was game to try and sort something out. Although most of the Harmsworth's work was with dogs and cats, more and more exotics were coming through the doors. We decided to make an anaesthetizing cage that would work for all manner of small animals, from birds to gerbils and hamsters. I found a transparent box, made of some kind of fairly solid perspex, in the store room. Trevor brought in his Black and Decker and made a hole in it, just big enough for the rubber tube that carried the gas.

'What on earth are you two doing?' Helen said, as she came into the prep room that afternoon.

'What does it look like?'

'An aquarium.'

'It's an anaesthetizing chamber for a budgerigar,' said Trevor with a justifiable degree of pride in his handiwork.

His remark got the required look of amazement. 'All that for a budgie? What's wrong with it?'

'A growth on the wing,' I said. 'Probably cancerous.'

'Sounds interesting. Need any help?'

The operation was listed for the following Monday, when I was the only one in the operating theatre. I had secretly been hoping that Tony Self would be so intrigued by the new equipment that he would suggest doing it himself. But he had let it be known that he would be busy in his office all day with paperwork. Any thoughts I might have had about postponing Beaky's op till another time were dashed when Magda put her head round the prep-room door. 'Helen tells me you're sorting out Flo's budgie this morning. Knew you wouldn't let me down.'

None the less, I left Beaky right till the end of the list.

He turned out to be particularly vicious. Not for the first time I wondered why people had budgies as pets. Eventually he was persuaded to enter the anaesthetic chamber, though only after taking a chunk out of my finger. Then, once the top was safely in place, Helen started pumping the gas in. Within minutes Beaky was unsteady on his pins, then finally keeled over and lay on his side. In a flash Helen had him out and attached to the huge anaesthetic tube via an adapter and a little home-made mask which Trevor had made out of plastic.

213

I grabbed hold of the growth and gave it a gentle tug to see what it was attached to. To my astonishment I felt it peel away completely, to leave a small wound which hardly bled at all and needed just one stitch, a job that was much less complicated than sewing on a button. Helen, who was concentrating on monitoring the anaesthetic, had not even seen what I was doing.

'Operation over nurse,' I said with mock pomposity. 'You can let the patient come round now. Give him pure oxygen.' In the meantime I had hidden the growth under a drape.

'How did you do that?' was her amazed reply.

'Oh it was nothing. I do it all the time.'

I turned round to write up the notes, leaving Helen to turn off the anaesthetic and give Beaky pure oxygen, and pondered how best to describe the way that the growth had more or less fallen off without actually making it look as if the whole exercise was totally unnecessary.

In the meantime Helen busied herself clearing up the array of instruments which had turned out to be completely redundant. I looked at the clock: twenty to one. No point in doing anything else this morning. Trevor and I and a couple of the nurses, including Helen, had arranged to go out to lunch at a local restaurant. Mrs Purser always had Mondays off. With a bit of luck we would get a whole hour in, I thought.

Yes, all in all, I decided, a good morning's work. The anaesthetic chamber had worked perfectly and Beaky could be returned as good as new to Flo. No deaths on my conscience, feathered or otherwise. Time to get Beaky back in his cage. I picked it up from the floor and put it on the operating table.

But where was he? Helen was busy packing up the instruments. 'Let's be having him then,' I said.

Still Practising

'What do you mean?'

'Beaky the budgie.'

'Didn't you put him back?' Helen asked with a look of amused exasperation on her face. My bouts of absent-mindedness were becoming well known.

'No.' A sudden wave of panic enveloped me. Helen saw that I wasn't joking and suddenly I wasn't the only one panicking. She had taken her eyes off the patient having put him on pure oxygen, not anticipating any problems in his recovery. There was no doubt about it: the bird had flown.

We began to act like demented chickens ourselves, looking for him in ridiculous places, under the instruments tray, under the table. Absolutely no sign.

'Whatever you do don't open the door,' I said, sounding like Captain Mainwaring from *Dad's Army*.

'Thank God the windows are shut,' Helen added. 'At least he can't have gone far.'

We searched high and low all over the operating theatre, but to no avail.

'Listen!' Helen said suddenly. We stopped in our tracks and stayed perfectly still. Then I heard it too, a faint chirping sound. It stopped and then about twenty seconds later started again. 'He's flown up the anaesthetic tube!' said Helen.

I put my ear to the corrugated rubber hose. Halfway up I could hear the faint chirping of a slightly squiffy budgie. 'Now what are we going to do?' I could hear the desperation in my voice. It wasn't the health of the budgie that worried me, he would come to no harm – he was breathing pure oxygen by now. No, it was the expensive anaesthetic tube I was worried about.

I could see there was no option but to cut it up into little slices to get Beaky out. Out of the corner of my eye, through the glass pane of the operating-room door, I could see Tony Self chatting to Mary in the corridor. I could only pray that he didn't come in now.

Neither of us said a word. Then Helen decided to lift the cage up high and stuff the end of the tube into the door in the vain hope that, like hot air, the budgie would rise. To encourage him to go along with this plan, I gently shook the bottom end of the tube. I was just about to give up and get the scalpel blade out to start hacking bits off when there was a rapid fluttering of wings and Beaky appeared at the bottom of the cage. He stumbled out, saw his perch and hopped onto it, looking none the worse for wear. Quick as a flash Helen had the cage door shut and had just taken the tube out as the boss walked in.

'So, how did it go?' he asked. He'd been following our Heath Robinson DIY with interest – though from a distance.

'Fine – er – I think. After a bit of excitement,' I added, not planning to go into details unless I could help it. But he wasn't listening, he was bending down, peering through the bars of Beaky's cage.

'Hmmm. Nice neat job, David – and a good recovery. You'll have to become our budgie expert!'

I looked at him and wondered if he knew what he was saying. But how could he? He couldn't know about Duncan, could he?

When I told Andy later, he told me it was called a Pyrrhic victory, which is to say a victory you would rather not have won.

Magda of course was delighted. ''Ow d'ya fancy a trip to Lime'ouse, darlin'? You're not on duty tonight, I've checked with the roster. I'll be dropping back about 6.30 when I come to pick up me chara. So see you then.'

Still Practising

As I said, Magda was a battler. How could I refuse? At 6.30 sharp I climbed into her 'chara' – short for charabanc, she explained later, an old Commer van that had had windows cut in the back some years before to save on purchase tax, she explained. It had two bench seats, one facing the front in the usual way and one facing the back, which passengers got into from the double doors at the rear. She had got the seats, she said, from a scrap yard. It didn't surprise me. There were no seat belts in those days, but Magda had rigged up an intriguing system of hooked elasticated straps, known as bungies, to keep animal cages from sliding all over the place. Humans just had to rely on their size keeping them firmly wedged in. Magda confided that when she had four up in the back, she'd make sure she had a thin one with a fat one, 'to stop them rattlin' around'. Fortunately there were no other passengers that night, and I sat in the front seat.

Flo lived in a red brick block that must have been more than a hundred years old. If it hasn't been knocked down, her flat would now be worth a fortune, as it was right on the Thames, looking across the river to the wharves at Rotherhithe. Not that we went there directly. We made two stops, one to drop off a bag of groceries and the other to pick up a bag of washing.

Magda gave three hearty knocks on Flo's door, then without waiting for a reply, got out a key and went in. The key ring that it was attached to had another forty or so keys on it. 'Are those . . . ?'

'Yea,' she replied. 'I know, I know. Barkin', ain't I?'

Flo's flat smelled of mildew and gas fire. The old lady herself was sitting by the window. Outside I could see the lights of riverboats reflected in the water.

''Ow many times have I told you to draw them curtains

217

when it gets dark Flo?' These windows let in the draughts somefing terrible,' she said, then turning her attention to me, 'Now Flo, guess who I've brought to see you.'

'No idea.'

The old lady was wearing a hairnet and was a dead ringer for Ena Sharples, the old battleaxe of Coronation Street, with manners to match.

At that point Magda put her finger to her lips, walked over to where I was holding the cage and whipped off the cover. ''Allo. 'Allo. Give us a puff. Give us a puff.'

I nearly jumped out of my skin. Houdini couldn't have planned it better. Although budgies do talk if you get them young enough, Beaky had never said a word throughout his ordeal. It must have been the overpowering smell of cigarette smoke that told him he was back home.

'Beaky!' Flo's voice had lost the hard edge of a moment back and I could see in her the shy young girl posing in the sepia photograph with her handsome, smiling young man about to set off for the trenches.

Magda opened the cage door and Beaky flew to the old lady's outstretched arm. 'We can't stay long, Flo, but I thought you'd like to meet the young vet 'ere who put Beaky to rights. This is Mr Grant.'

Flo looked up at me, her mouth smiling, her eyes completely clouded over. It was only then that I realized she was blind. 'Did you say Grant, Magda?'

'Nuffink wrong with your 'earing, Flo. So, go on then, say thank you, you silly old woman, while I make us all a cuppa.'

'Hope he ain't caused you no trouble,' Flo said when we were all sitting down and Beaky was helping himself to some crumbs from the cake that Magda had brought with her.

'No trouble at all,' I said, looking at the plaster on my

right hand where Beaky had vented his anger, which was even now stained with blood.

''Cos 'e can be a real terror.' Beaky was now helping himself to my cake. I decided not to pick it up, but let him take his fill. 'Is your Mr Grant comin' to the Christmas knees-up Magda?'

Magda turned to look at me, with an expression I last saw on the face of the Cub Mistress when I said I didn't know how to boil an egg. 'I don't think he'd miss it for anyfing. Would you darlin'?'

I had heard how in the summer Magda organised at least one outing to the seaside. That summer she had hired a coach and taken her old dears to Margate. With her usual persuasive powers she was helped by some of the hospital nurses. This was obviously the Christmas equivalent, I realized.

Magda asked if I would mind if we stopped off in Hackney on our way back to Finsbury Park. She had some animals to feed, she said. She led the way down the side of a beautiful Victorian villa set back from a dilapidated garden square, where once nannies must have sat next to upholstered perambulators. The area had been badly bombed in the war and this square was an oasis in a forest of tower blocks. As for the garden in the centre, it was now taken up with two very nasty looking prefabs.

Two cats were sitting on the window ledge and as soon as Magda turned the key, a cacophony of barking began and we were both nearly knocked down as a variety of animals hurled themselves at us.

'They seem to know you really well,' I said.

'They should do, this is where I live,' Magda laughed.

It turned out that she had four dogs and five cats, all of them animals who had failed to be homed and who would otherwise have had to be put down. She was always coming across other hopeless cases and had to be persuaded not to take any more on.

'That's the great thing about basement flats, the garden.' She walked over to the back, and when she opened the door the dogs immediately rushed out. It was large for London and walled all the way round in pale brown brick, a good 80 feet long and wider than usual, as these houses had been quite elegant in their day.

'And we've got Victoria park about five minutes' walk away for the dogs. And there's no traffic here, so the cats come and go as they please, so don't you go thinkin' you'll call the RSPCA and be havin' me up for cruelty,' she chortled.

Soon we were back in the 'chara' heading for the Harmsworth. The buses were 'somefing terrible', she said. She wouldn't hear of not taking me back.

'So I'll put you down for the Christmas do then shall I? I've laid on a conjurer this year and a drag queen. It'll be a real good laugh.'

'Isn't a drag queen a bit . . . er . . . ,' I hesitated, searching for the right phrase, 'close to the knuckle?' I suggested.

'Close to the knuckle?' she repeated in amazement. 'You must be jokin'. These lot were watching drag when Danny La Rue was still in nappies, darlin'. All dressed up like a dogs' dinner – they love it.'

'Now, I know what you're thinking,' she continued without taking breath. 'But don't you worry about takin' time off. Tony is always very accommodating. And bein' as you're so strong, you'll be handy for the wheelchairs. Tell you somefing' darlin',' she added, as we pulled into the Harmsworth car park. 'If I was twenty years younger . . .' And with that she blew me a kiss, and drove off into the night.

Chapter Fifteen

Gloria was determined to continue my South American education. Although London was not as cosmopolitan in the early seventies as it is now, there were a handful of restaurants known to the South American community. I remember two in particular that Gloria introduced me to. One was a Mexican place in Chelsea. Going there was not just about the superb food, it was the whole Mexican experience; the atmosphere was like nothing I had come across before, especially the live music. The regular singer was a statuesque Mexican woman, all fiery eyes and curling mouth, with a voice that could be provocative one moment and soft and romantic the next, and there was always a brilliant guitar accompaniment. It was hearing the wonderful singing in Andalucia on holiday with Keith (and not being able to understand what they were singing about) that had made me want to learn Spanish in the first place. And here I was, listening and understanding – well, beginning to.

You didn't need to have a whole meal, and I used to go there regularly just to hear her sing. My favourite song was not Mexican at all, but Chilean: *'En de Que Te Vi'* about a man who falls in love at first sight. And a lullaby from Cuba, *'Duerme Negrito'*, was guaranteed to put a lump in my throat: about a poor *campesina* singing to her baby while his father was slaving in the sugar-cane fields for a pittance.

The other restaurant Gloria took me to was Paraguayan, and was in Beauchamp Place. It had a band featuring a Paraguayan harp. The four-course meal would last all evening but nobody cared – the music was so wonderful the waiters would have to remind their customers to eat. As for the Grant classical music collection, for the time being it was put on hold. What I wanted now was anything and everything South American.

But I was dreading Christmas. Although Gloria wasn't a girlfriend in the conventional sense, I had got used to doing things with her and when she told me she was going back to Colombia for two weeks I was knocked sideways. Not only would I have no Caroline, but now no Gloria. And, worst of all, no one to spend New Year's Eve with. How wrong can one be!

Magda was like a London taxi, unstoppable except at her command. And command was the word on the night of the old folks' party. She was like a general. Most function rooms in pubs were upstairs and it had taken some time to find one on the ground floor with wheelchair access. It was a large Edwardian gin palace in Bethnal Green. The bar could have been in a museum, with floor-to-ceiling gilt mirrors and mahogany you could see your face in. It was called the Three Fiddlers.

'All bloody fiddlers, if you ask me, mate,' Vic, a former docker, informed me as I brought a pint of special to the table where I had put his wheelchair. 'All that froff,' he said, flicking the beer with his finger. 'What do they call this, Babycham? They must be making a packet out of us lot. What do they fink we are, blind or somefink?'

'Don't you take no notice, lad,' his friend Arthur gave my arm a nudge. 'As for you Vic, you should fink yourself lucky you can have a bloody pint. Old Alf whatsisname, can't even hold a pint glass his hand it shakes so much. 'Ere,' he said, turning to me again. 'What's your name?

'David.'

'Right, David, do us a favour will ya, get us another one in before the entertainment starts?'

Magda was right: nothing would faze this lot, I decided. They had lived through two world wars and they would live through anything life threw at them. If a stripper had come on I wouldn't have been surprised.

The ratio of old folks to helpers was about two to one. Although we had to pay for our food – 'turkey and all the trimmings' – it was worth it just to see these old-timers enjoying themselves.

Flo was there, dressed up to the nines in green satin, grey hair tightly permed, hairnet nowhere to be seen. I went up and introduced myself and asked after my former patient. Beaky was doing well, she said. The man from the council who had come to mend the Ascot water heater in the bathroom had refused to come in unless Beaky was in his cage. Which was just as it should be, she said. He was clearly back on form. 'I could've frottled him meself when I got done up t'night,' she said. 'See these sparklers?' and she fingered the necklace around her throat. 'Blow me if he didn't start peckin' at 'em. Like they was seed. Like as not he could see hisself in 'em. He went straight in 'is cage, I can tell ya. No messin'.'

'How do you get him to go in?' I asked, remembering that Flo couldn't see.

'Trainin',' Flo decided after a second or two's pause.

'Magda,' I said when I found her leaning behind the bar, trying to have a quiet smoke, as the party was winding down. 'When Flo said she was wearing her sparklers, did she mean, you know, sparklers . . . er . . . diamonds?'

'Brains as well as brawn I see. You'll go far,' she replied stubbing out her cigarette and preparing to sound the retreat to the troops.

'I mean, do you suppose they are real diamonds?'

She motioned me aside and lowered her voice. 'Name Harry Fountain mean anything?'

I said it did ring a vague bell, but I couldn't think where.

'Local villain. According to Flo he was the Reggie Kray of the twenties. Ran a boxing gym. His manor stretched from Stepney right through Bethnal Green. Didn't do him much good though. Did fifteen years in Dartmoor for manslaughter then popped it two months before he was due for release.'

I wasn't sure how to respond to that: righteous affront or compassion. I imagine that what flashed across my face was more compassion than indignation because Magda soon chipped in. 'I know what you're thinking, but don't. Flo says she was never so relieved as when she got the call. After five years she'd taken up with a geezer as ran a garage in Limehouse. Had two kids by 'im and never said a word. They were bloody terrified when the parole came through.'

'So the sparklers?'

'She'd had them all the time. Hidden in the Ascot, she said. Everything else was taken when Harry went down.'

'By the police?'

'The old bill had nuffink to do with it. Some heavies from Leyton, Flo said. Turned the place over. But not well enough.'

'But they must be worth a fortune . . .'

'That's as may be. But they're worth more to Flo around her neck on nights like this. They give her "respect". Everyone knows they're the real thing. Don't forget, David, this is the East End. Without her sparklers Flo is just a blind old lady on her uppers. With them she's Flo Fountain, widow of Harry Fountain, cockney legend. Respect, David. It's all about respect.'

The evening ended with a sing-song, with another old bird on the piano, thumping them out like there was no tomorrow: 'Roll Out the Barrel', 'My Old Man Said Follow the Van' and others I didn't know. Those that still had use of their legs joined hands and were giving it, as Magda would say, a lot of welly.

On New Year's Eve I had two invitations, one to a dance hosted by the university athletics club and the other a black-tie do thrown by a Colombian friend of Henry's. There was no competition. I had spent Christmas Day back in Rochester and, just as I suspected, my dinner jacket was still hanging in my wardrobe smelling of the mothballs put there by my mother, and luckily the dress shirt I had bought when I was nineteen still did up, though only just.

The party was in Holland Park, London at its poshest. It was a huge, double-fronted house with torches marking the entrance and a section of the road outside was roped off by police to allow cars to pull up. Fortunately I had arranged with Henry to meet him at the Bar Galicia at nine, from where it was only a five-minute walk. Berta had decided to stay at home with Alejandro. Neither Henry nor I had thought to bring the printed invitation and getting in without it was like getting through immigration without a passport. The maitre d', with the manners of a sergeant major, asked for our names and scanned the guest lists, which ran to several pages. As I followed his eyes, I caught the name Picasso among others.

'Surely not *the* Picasso?' I said to Henry in a half-whisper, scanning the guests for a shiny bald head and a big nose. This would be something to tell the boys upstairs, I thought. It had become a habit to drop in on them when I got back. If Andy wasn't there to improve me, then Roy was always good for a laugh, with stories that made my hair curl. All the while Bill would sit there, gently smiling to himself.

'Oh no, the old boy is far too old and wouldn't dream of leaving his patch in the south of France. Some of his far-flung children no doubt. A couple of them are about the right age and live in Paris. It's probably them.'

I was beginning to get worried. Unfortunately the names were not in alphabetical order and there seemed to be pages of them. Then suddenly from the top of the stairs a voice rang out. It was Henry's friend, our host. All it took was a nod and, champagne glasses in our hands, we were through the rope barrier and up the massive staircase which took up half the front of the house. Then Henry was off, hugging and *hola*-ing. From upstairs came the sound of salsa. From another room, I could hear two guitars. Everyone seemed to glitter, and I couldn't help remembering Flo and her sparklers. They wouldn't be out of place here I thought.

'David!' I turned at the sound of my English name amid the hubbub of Spanish, and recognized José, one of Henry's brothers. 'Come and meet a friend of mine.' He turned to a young woman with softly curling dark brown hair streaked with gold. '*Doña* Gloria, meet David Grant, a friend and colleague of Henry's.'

Another Gloria! And why the unusual '*Doña*'? Before I could come to any conclusions the *doña* had extended a very pretty hand covered with gold rings. What was I supposed to do? It didn't look as if it was intended to be shaken, so I lifted it to my lips in what I hoped looked like a practised manner.

She was utterly gorgeous, like an exotic flower you

might find in a hothouse, with velvet skin and a flawless complexion, and she was so slight I felt I could have lifted her up with one hand but was frightened of bruising her. Although she was wearing extremely high heels, her head barely reached my chest. The eyes looking up at me were so dark and deep I felt they could watch me without giving anything away – as if she were wearing sunglasses.

'David, I hope you don't mind, but I have to go and find my wife, she's wandered off somewhere. I wonder if I could ask you to look after *Doña* Gloria for me.'

I gave José a Cary Grant-style leave-it-to-me tilt of the chin and turned to my companion. 'Are you from Colombia?' How pathetic.

'Do you know it?'

'Unfortunately not.' A pause. Then I tried again. 'Do you come from the same region as José and Henry?'

'No? Santander.'

'But isn't that on the north coast of Spain?'

That was the first time I heard her tinkling laugh.

'Yes, my late husband's family came from there originally, but many, many years ago. Centuries I think. But there is a region of Colombia that is called Santander, but rather hot, not very pleasant, far from the coast. The family has a *finca* there, but we rarely go. And of course it is nothing like the north coast of Spain, which has a wonderful climate. Many noble Spanish families have their summer residences there. Do you know it?'

But I was still thinking about the first part of what she said. Late husband. How good was her command of English? Did she mean that he hadn't arrived at the party yet, or that he had died? I have to admit that I hoped it was the latter. But then what about the 'we'?

It seemed bizarre, but also appropriate, that the two

most glamorous women I had ever met were both called Gloria. Very suitable. Gloria No. 2 was quite different from Gloria No. 1, however. Gloria 1 was tall and elegant, with straight black hair, whereas Gloria 2 was small and vivacious and spoke in an excitable way that I discovered was quite normal for many Latinas and particularly those who come from Medellin, which I later learned was where she grew up. And whereas Gloria 1 and I always spoke Spanish, Gloria 2 and I hardly ever did. José had introduced us in English and it stayed that way.

I wondered how I could find out more about her. Meanwhile I had to discuss the weather in Spain. But it was a start – it hadn't done Eliza Doolittle any harm. 'No, *Doña* Gloria, I know the south coast a little, but not the north I'm afraid.' I wasn't about to mention Torremelinos. 'Though I have heard the mountains are very nice. For walking.' I finished lamely.

'Poofff,' she said, an untranslatable explosion of sound that I would get to know well. 'I hate walking. But,' she added, her eyes glinting, 'I love dancing.' Then, picking a bit of fluff off the lapel of my dinner jacket, she went on, narrowing her eyes. 'Do you like to salsa, David?'

I couldn't believe my luck! Over the past few weeks since that first party, I had had a number of opportunities to shake a leg, as Magda would say. 'Not very well, Dona, but . . .' and the debonair Cary Grant persona I had nurtured for the past five minutes gave way to keen-as-mustard John Travolta.

'That is what I love about you English,' and I shivered as she touched my arm again. 'No stupid pride. Pride in general is a much overrated virtue I think, don't you? In fact I don't consider it a virtue at all. Far too many of my ancestors lost their lives because of their pride. Well then, what are we waiting for?' She took my hand and soon we were practically running along the corridor to the back of the house where the music was coming from.

'Oh and no more of this *Doña* nonsense,' she added, turning her head as we hurried along. 'It is only José's little joke because my father is rich and José likes to embarrass me. Call me Gloria.'

And I did.

That night the music and the champagne (French, not Spanish or South American) – not to mention the beautiful people – were too much for a frustrated grammar-school boy to resist and I discovered that salsa was not just a dance, with steps and movements to be learned and practised till they were perfect, it was the most seductive and passionate introduction to romance that could be imagined.

From the moment I met Gloria all thoughts of Caroline and her 28-year old girl's blouse of a tutor disappeared – for a few hours at least. On the odd occasions that I became aware of my surroundings rather than my partner, I had fleeting glimpses of famous faces, so fleeting that I found I usually couldn't put a name to them, except Bianca Jagger, who was unmistakeable and seemed to be there without her husband. Just before midnight the word went out that there were flamenco dancers in another room. And, eyes sparkling, we went up and watched the smouldering sensual circling of a man and a woman. Castanets clicked, guitars strummed rhythmically and a man sitting on a chair sang – although it sounded more like a wail. Gloria stood in front of me and I leant my head on hers as we watched. Then on the stroke of midnight she turned round and lifted her head to mine.

'*Feliz año nuevo!*' she said, her face turned upwards towards me. And I bent down and kissed her, and I remember thinking, I wonder what Schopenhauer would have to say about this – though not for long.

Although New Year's Day was not a bank holiday, there were no operations set for the morning, and for some strange reason we had hardly any patients that afternoon. How did the animals know not to be ill, I wondered. However this state of affairs was quite usual apparently and there was just a skeleton staff on duty.

Among those who did turn up was Dolly Harding with Whisky. I had seen them before Christmas. Whisky was a black cat who was always fighting. Although he had been castrated some years before, he had learned his trade thoroughly and was not about to forget it. Whisky was the terror of the neighbourhood and had the scars to prove it. He had had a nasty abscess on his back, where a bite from another local tearaway had become infected. I had sent him on his way with an injection of antibiotic.

For my trouble Dolly had insisted on giving me a brand new electric kettle. The policy of the Harmsworth was that people would give what they could, and there was a collection box in reception. But occasionally we would be given things, not money. Bridey Donovan, for example, usually had a poem in her handbag which she would first recite and then give to me.

I had decided that as the flat belonged to the Harmsworth, and it didn't have an electric kettle, there would be no harm in accepting it.

'You said as I should bring Whisky back for a check up,' she said to remind me, although I hardly needed any reminding. It was not every day I was given a brand new kettle as a thank you.

'Right Mrs Harding. Let's be having him, then.'

She lifted the basket onto the examining table. The wound was healing nicely I noticed.

'He looks fine. Eating all right is he? Bowels all right?'

'Oh yes. Never better, which is why I bought you this. I thought you might be in need.' From a large holdall, she took out an electric kettle and proffered it to me.

I was so stunned I took it; it was exactly the same as the first kettle. 'But Mrs Harding . . .' I hesitated. 'You have already given me a kettle. Last time you were here. And I have been using it and it's been extremely useful.'

'You can't have too many kettles, that's what I say. You never know when they're going to go wrong, do you. And then where would you be?'

'But I can't take it Mrs Harding.'

'Why not? The sign out the front says give what you can, and this is what I can. I can give this kettle. I don't need it. Think of it as a Christmas present.'

'But it's brand new.'

Of course it is. I wouldn't palm you off with any old rubbish.'

There was nothing to do but to accept it. There was sure to be somewhere it could go: the nurse's day room, or the kitchen: Mrs Purser could probably do with it.

'By the way,' I said when I saw Trevor getting into his car to set off back to Muswell Hill, 'do you need a kettle, by any chance?'

'Oh, Dolly Harding was in was she?'

'Yes, how did you know?'

'I just guessed. No. Just put it in the nurses' room, the cupboard next to the door.'

I went and collected the kettle and took it upstairs. Gill was there reading a magazine. 'Trevor said I should put this in a cupboard.'

She pointed to the right. 'That one.'

I opened the door and to my astonishment discovered it was filled with electric kettles exactly like the one I was holding in my hand, and the one that was even now sitting in my kitchen.

'Where does she get them?' I asked in bewilderment. 'Are they stolen?'

Gill shrugged. 'Nobody's ever plucked up the courage to find out. And anyway, they're useful, like Dolly says. It's surprising how they go, you know, wedding presents and so on.'

I had never been close to a parrot before, let alone had to examine one. So I was completely at sea when Mrs Lamb brought one in towards the end of surgery. For someone with such a mild-sounding surname she was very abrasive. It seemed she had brought him in before. 'Don't know what you're doing. I wouldn't give a rabbit's fart for the lot of you.'

This attitude was something I was getting to grips with. In Kent the clientele, from farmers to pet owners, had generally been polite and reasonable; exceptions were very few and far between.

It seemed that over recent weeks Mrs Lamb had been seen by both Trevor (who at least knew something about parrots and had an interest in them) and by the boss. This parrot, who was called Pedro, was always supposed to be 'under the weather': he was 'off his food' she insisted, although examinations had never found any problem.

'I want tests,' she insisted. 'I want to know what's wrong with 'im.'

But what tests? I didn't have a clue. Mrs Lamb sat on the one available chair and looked as if she wouldn't budge until I had come up with something positive.

At least things weren't busy for once, and I nipped next door to Trevor. 'See if you can't persuade her to have him admitted. At least we can keep an eye on him and see for ourselves if he eats normally.'

'Right Mrs Lamb,' I said when I returned. 'The first thing we need to do is to have him in. Then we can give him the tests in a sterile environment.'

As I had already learned in Canterbury, the scientific approach can work wonders. She agreed. 'At long last someone who's prepared to do somefing,' she harrumphed. 'But I'm warning you, I'm not having him back till you're sure 'e's better.'

In 1971 the Harmsworth did not have a dedicated exotics ward and so Pedro was put in Ward 4 which doubled up at the time as the exotics ward, along with a few other assorted inmates: a guinea pig with mange, some stray pet mice, a hamster, a healthy stray Siamese cat waiting to be rehomed, and another African grey parrot which had been with us for a week, having strayed from home, and which so far had not been claimed. He had arrived just after Christmas and had been the picture of misery from the beginning. He had been subdued all week and hadn't said a word that might have given us a clue where he came from.

'That African grey,' I said to Trevor later down at the pub.

'Oh, you mean Pedro.'

'No the other one in Ward 4. Well when I took Pedro in to join him, he seemed to perk up.'

'Could be. Well, if Pedro can get him to talk we might have something to go on. Even his name would help.'

There was nothing wrong with the parrot, Trevor said,

David Grant

and adverts were being placed in various places to let people know where he was but without even a name it was hopeless. And also Christmas was a difficult time when nothing was routine.

We decided to keep Pedro in for some time. Not only might he be good for the unknown parrot, we decided, but the unknown parrot might be good for Pedro.

Although Mrs Lamb continued to pester the hospital with daily calls, we could quite honestly tell her that Pedro was doing very well. In fact he was positively thriving. There was always someone either working in the ward or popping in to check on the animals and he seemed to love the company. He took to one of the nurses, Janine, in particular, bobbing up and down and screeching with joy whenever she came in.

'Probably just bored. Simple as that,' said Tony Self on one of his daily ward rounds.

'I bet he's left on his own for a good part of the day. At least in here there's lots going on, and with that one here as well,' he added, indicating the stray parrot, 'he's got one of his kind to talk to.'

And talk was indeed the word. A couple of days later Janine went into the ward to say hello to Pedro. The attention he gave her had worked in the same way it does for humans – she was as taken with him as he was with her. He did his usual bobbing about and then suddenly from behind her Janine heard a strong Scottish voice say, 'You f****** b*******!' It was the stray African grey, who far from bobbing up and down with joy seemed to be bobbing up and down with fury, annoyed by all the attention Pedro was getting.

'That's a bit rude,' said Janine, turning to look at the stray bird.

' Gi' us a whisky.' This time the strong Scottish accent was even more unmistakeable.

This certainly narrowed the field in terms of the identity of its owner down. A Scot. But living in London, or north of the border? We needed more information, and with Janine's help we hoped the parrot could be coaxed to say more and more. The next day, seeing the Siamese cat being fed, he came out with 'Eat it all up or you'll get a smack', which after my recent experience of Adam and Tracy, I didn't feel like laughing at.

What was interesting was that it was only when Janine was around that any talking went on. Perhaps his owner was a 5 foot 6 inch blonde with a Marc Bolan-style haircut, I surmised, just like Janine. Soon one of the very bright young nurses worked out that if you knocked on the door and didn't go in, he would imagine it was Janine and would start talking to tempt her in. Two days later, in a perfect Scottish brogue, he came out with his name (Hamish, hardly a surprise) and his address, somewhere near St Albans.

'Vocabulary's a bit choice, isn't it?' said Tony to his owners a few days later when they arrived to claim him. Trevor and I had taken bets that one of them would have the T Rex haircut, but no. There was no doubt as to the owner-ship, however. Hamish had got his owner's voice off to perfection.

'He was clearly very defensive when it came to the ripe language,' said Tony, who spoke to them. 'He said that the bird had only to hear something once and that was it. Although when I asked how many years they had lived in St Albans, that didn't quite square with his account of a plumber having provided the vocabulary. Not many Scottish plumbers in St Albans, I imagine. He said he'd "tried to train him out of it" but had failed. At least I was able to end on a more positive note. I told him how Hamish had helped another parrot we had in here.'

And indeed, Mrs Lamb had come to collect Pedro the day before. The fact that he bucked right up just from seeing Hamish had proved to us, at least, that there was nothing wrong with him. He returned to his owner with a clean bill of health – by the time he left he had the appetite of a horse.

But that wasn't quite the end of the parrot saga. At lunchtime the next day Tony came down to tell us he had just had a call from a very irate Mrs Lamb. 'She was absolutely furious,' he said, waving his cigarette holder in the air. 'Wanted to know the name of the Scotsman on our staff. Said he should be sacked. Said she would be writing to Head Office about the kind of people we employ.'

It seemed that the choice vocabulary of our Scottish visitor had been picked up by Pedro, and he had taken to insulting his owner throughout the day. And when he wasn't doing that he was mewing like a Siamese cat. It seemed that we would not be seeing Mrs Lamb and her parrot again.

For the next few days, as the story travelled, the whole hospital was ringing with various attempts to master a Scottish accent. By far and away the most irritating was Trevor, who spent the next few days talking to me in the most terrible fake Scottish accent. What he didn't realize was that it was really very good and reminded me of Duncan.

I had taken to dropping in to chat with whoever was on night duty when I got back to the flat after an evening out. It was a nice way to wind down. But I hadn't been in since New Year's Eve.

'A new girl is it?' Bill said as soon as he saw my face at the door.'

'How did you guess?'

Just then a call came in and I made for the door. I really wasn't up to chit-chat tonight.

'Pass me my indigestion pills will you David?' Bill said, his hand over the phone. 'That's the trouble with Christmas, too much eating and Phyllis, she does know how to push the boat out.' He looked even more like Father Christmas than usual this evening, I thought, with his ever-growing belly pushing out a brand new red v-necked lamb's wool jumper.

'By the way, Gloria called.'

'Gloria?'

'That's right. Said you'd call her back.'

'Thanks Bill, I will.'

Gloria called. But which one? If I'd heard the voice then I would know, they were so different. But what should I do now? This was a delicate matter that called for analysis and skill, if not cunning. Gloria 1 was a friend. If it wasn't her, I wouldn't be risking anything if I called her. I could easily say it was an old message I had picked up. But if I called Gloria 2 and it wasn't her, I might even blow it.

She had gone to Paris for a few days and had said she would call me on her return. But I couldn't call her if she hadn't called me.

So I phoned Gloria 1. She had got back from Colombia earlier that week. The phone rang and rang. Blast. There were no answering machines in 1971. I would just have to wait. But what if it was Gloria 2? If I didn't call she would think it was incredibly rude. Andy would have an answer, but unfortunately he was not on duty.

When I got to my flat I called down to Bill.

'What did you tell her?'

'Who?'

'Gloria.'

'Oh. That I'd give you the message that she'd called.'

'Did you tell her I was out?'

'I can't rightly remember David, but I expect so. Because you were.'

'Right.'

'She was in a call box.'

'A call box?'

'Yes. In the airport, I think she said.'

'Thank you Bill, thank you very much!'

It was Gloria 2.

I looked at my watch. Eleven o'clock. Too late to call now anyway, I decided. I went to sleep that night with a smile on my face.

Chapter Fifteen

The prospectus for the bone-fixing conference in Davos arrived later that week. While other people in the Harmsworth were poring over holiday brochures and dreaming of beaches, I was drooling over courses on fixing bones – though the photographs of snow-covered mountains did not escape my notice. It looked even more exciting than I had imagined, but after a look at the small print – the price – I began to realize what an uphill job it would be persuading Tony to let me go. I would just have to convince him that the hospital would benefit once this young, enthusiastic and talented young colleague began revolutionizing the way we handled fractures. There was no point putting it off, I decided, and with the adrenalin still flowing, I went to beard him in his den.

As Tony looked over the prospectus, his cigarette for once abandoned on the edge of an ashtray, I gave a running commentary about how much of our work concerned broken bones and how much it seemed to me that this new way of working would help by cutting down the nursing time, not to mention enhancing the reputation of the Harmsworth.

'I take your point, David. No doubt about that. The only problem as I see it, and as sure as God made little green apples it is a problem, is money.' It wasn't just the cost of the course, he explained, but the costs involved in setting up the new system. 'But look, leave it with me and I'll see what

I can do. Mind you, I can't promise anything. Depends whether I can persuade the finance committee that this isn't some jolly enabling you to learn to ski.'

A couple of days later I was summoned to his office. He looked a bit uncomfortable and whatever hopes I might have been nursing over the past couple of days that I'd soon be breathing Swiss mountain air were dashed before he even opened his mouth. 'Sorry to disappoint you, David,' he said briskly, looking over his half-moon frames. 'But we won't be able to send you on the orthopaedics course. I put it to the Chief Veterinary Officer and he says that it would be a jolly good idea for someone to go, however he rather thinks that in order to get finance, that someone should be me.'

I sat the other side of his desk expressionless, but inside I was completely dumbfounded, I opened my mouth to say, 'But I found the course!', but no words came out.

'As sure as God made little green apples,' Tony continued, 'if this proposal came in front of the committee with your name on it, they would veto it. The long and the short of it is that you just haven't been here long enough, David. In essence it needs someone with more experience. I'm sorry.'

'Bloody cheek,' I said later, venting my spleen to Trevor over a pint. 'I mean, I found the bloody thing. If I hadn't been interested, hadn't been looking, then he would never have heard about it!'

Trevor grinned. He was totally unsympathetic. 'There, there Maestro. He's the boss and you just have to do what you're told. Anyway if he does bring this system in it'll need more than T. Self, MRCVS, to put it into practice. Maybe you – or even we – could go next year. How about that? Cheer up. That gloomy expression does nothing for your pulling power.' He ducked as I aimed a cuff.

Still Practising

'At least it looks as if there won't be enough time to fit in any skiing,' I said. 'Now that I've had a good look at it, the timetable hardly leaves time to eat, let alone anything else.'

'Sour grapes,' laughed Trevor. 'Anyway we're not all sporty types like you. Can you see the boss skiing? I mean, where would he put his cigarette holder? The amount he smokes I doubt if at that altitude he'd be fit enough to do anything more than make it from the lecture theatre to the bar. I mean 2000 metres, that's high.'

'How on earth do you know that?'

Trevor sat back in his chair and grinned. 'I did a spot of research, in case they decided to send me instead. After all, I've been here longer than you.'

I aimed another mistimed blow and then laughed it off. Tony was probably right, I reflected later. A junior vet would not carry as much clout as he would.

In the meantime I had Gloria to console me, and for the next few weeks I felt like a butterfly that had emerged from a chrysalis. I had money in my pocket and someone to spend it on.

Doña Gloria was a woman who knew what she liked: good food, good music, good fun. For sheer stamina, I was left standing; Gloria could party to the small hours night after night. One particular evening I remember started at the Bar Galicia and ended up in a flat in Mayfair at four in the morning. I found I was drinking just to stay awake. And then at some point I must have passed out – or, as I put it to the boss when I saw him the next morning, gone to sleep. Although living above the shop it wasn't a question of turning up in the clothes I had been wearing the night before, no amount of clean shirts and aftershave could disguise the fact that I was in a terrible state. I could hardly walk, my legs didn't feel as though they were part of my body. I had to think what to do with them: ah yes, this one forward, then shift the weight, pause. Now the same with the other one.

'Are you all right?' Tony said, as he passed me in the corridor.

'Er . . .'

'No. Clearly not. Touch of flu?'

'Er . . . Just overtired, I think. I didn't get home last night,' at which I decided that standing up was much easier if you were leaning against a wall. So I did.

'Go to bed David and do not come back before four o'clock.'

Those were the sweetest words I had heard all week. So I did what I was told, went upstairs, and crashed out.

At four o'clock I went down the back stairs out of the flat door and into Reception. Even though it was only an hour till the surgery closed, the waiting room was still full. A puppy was running around out of control, upsetting other animals which were either caged or quietly waiting with their owners. It also seemed to be limping. I went over and picked it up.

'Who does this dog belong to?' I asked, looking around me.

''Ere, you put 'im down,' came a voice from behind. I turned around to see a young woman, younger than me, stabbing her finger aggressively in the air.

I walked over and handed the puppy back to her. 'This dog should be on a lead, under control,' I continued.

'Don't you tell me what to do, mister. You keep your nose out of this,' she continued shouting after me as I went over to reception to check if I had any messages. 'And learn to mind your own bloody business!'

As I waited for the receptionist to finish a phone call I couldn't help but think of the contrast between Canterbury and here. What was even stranger was that in Canterbury they were paying and here our services were free. Funny old world.

'Mr Self wants you to take over from Mr Garcia,' the receptionist told me.

'Can't stand the pace, that's your trouble,' Henry told me with a smirk when I went in to relieve him a couple of minutes later. 'Though Gloria speaks highly of you.'

'Which one?'

'*La Doña* of course. Though I had a call from the other one yesterday. She wondered if you were all right. You haven't been returning her calls, she said. She didn't understand because you hadn't had a row or anything.'

I groaned. 'It's the boys in the backroom,' I said. 'They just give me a message that Gloria called and think that there's only one.'

'And you haven't told them any different I suppose?'

'I didn't want to confuse them.'

'Well, Granty, far be it from me to teach my grandfather to boil eggs, but I think you should sort it out. A woman scorned and all that . . .'

'I'm not scorning her.'

'Well, give her a call. Tell her about *La Doña*. I assume she doesn't know.'

'No.'

'Sometimes you just have to be brave, though of course it comes more naturally to us Latinos than to pasty-faced Englishmen.'

He successfully ducked the inevitable cuff. This was becoming a habit.

'So why do you all call her *La Doña*?'

'Just to rile her really. She's very rich you know. Nothing to do with her husband's family. They were just old blood, no money. No, it comes from her father, who is a very wealthy businessman. Textiles I think. Didn't she tell you?'

'Not in detail. She just said that her husband had been killed in a riding accident.'

The conversation ended when the nurse on duty handed me notes for the next client, a Mrs Norton. The door opened and the woman with the push-chair and the puppy came in.

'Oh,' she said. 'I didn't know you was the vet.'

I decided to say nothing. What was the point? She was feeling as uncomfortable as she was probably ever likely to feel as it was.

'Put him on the table, please.'

'I mean, if I'd known . . .'

'How did this happen?' I asked. No wonder the puppy was limping, he had several broken toes.

'A saucepan fell on him.'

'I see.'

'It's God's truth, so 'elp me.'

'It looks to me as if he was run over by something. I'll tell you again what I told you before. He needs to be kept on a lead, kept under control.'

I told her that her pet would have to be kept in for a few days. The foot would need to be set. Then I opened the door. 'That's all. You may go now.'

That night I decided to stay in. Bill and Andy were on duty, and I told them that if something came up that I could deal with, to let me know and not bother to call in whoever was officially on call.

But it was a quiet night. Another fox knocked down on the main Cambridge trunk road. He sounded as if he was too

Still Practising

badly injured to be brought back. Andy would have to put him down. Then there was a budgie who had flown behind the gas fire and wouldn't come out, somewhere over in Clapton. This was a surprisingly common occurrence and might need the Gas Board being called out, but they wouldn't go until the RSPCA had been there first.

Andy took off, leaving Bill and me discussing the night's intake so far. This wasn't the first time I had offered my services when I had nothing better to do. I found casualty work fascinating, trying out different shock treatments to see what worked best and sometimes sitting with an animal while it was on a drip watching for the seemingly miraculous response that a drip would often produce in a very ill animal.

While Bill took a sudden flurry of phone calls, I made a cup of tea and raided Mrs Purser's larder in the kitchen down the corridor to find a packet of biscuits.

'Thanks,' Bill said when I got back. 'Don't mind if I have one of these do you?' He had that characteristic sandpaper voice that comes from years of smoking. He took a cigarette paper from the packet by the phone and expertly distributed the tobacco and rolled it up. Roll-ups weren't as bad for you as the factory-made cigarettes, he told me. This particular bit of wisdom was trotted out every time he went into the ritual. And it had to be admitted, apart from the voice and a bit of a smoker's cough from time to time, he seemed to be as fit as a flea.

Andy radioed in. The fox was too far gone and he was going straight on to sort out the budgie. I decided I had had enough. Even with the extra hours' sleep I'd had courtesy of Tony, I still felt shattered. I was about to turn in when I noticed Bill holding his chest and grimacing in pain. He reached for some of the indigestion pills I'd seen him take

245

before.

'I've had this pain on and off for a couple of days now,' he managed to gasp. 'It just won't go.'

'You missus been feeding you up again has she, Bill?' I joked.

Then I looked at him. A sweat had broken out along his forehead.

The pain had obviously got a lot worse and he told me it was shooting down his left arm. What finally made me realize that something was really wrong was when the phone went and he didn't even try to reach for it but just lay back in the arm chair. 'I think I need a doctor,' he managed to blurt out.

I had come to the same conclusion and dialled 999, leaving the other phone ringing. They would just have to ring back.

Bill meanwhile had gone a deathly white colour and was beside himself with the pain. With immense relief I let the ambulance crew into the hospital ten minutes later. It all passed in a whirl after that and Bill was whisked off to hospital with the sirens blaring. He had managed to tell me his home phone number as they lifted him onto the stretcher and I phoned his wife letting her know where he was being treated so that she could go to his bedside. I had heard him talking to her so often on the phone, yet this was the first time I had heard her voice. Her son only lived in the next street, she said. I gave her the address of the hospital. Next I had to tell Andy. Fortunately I'd spent so much time in that room that I knew how to use the radio, and I got hold of him between calls to let him know what had happened. I would take all the calls until he got back, I told him.

I didn't have to wait long. The phone rang a few minutes

later; I looked at my watch – 1.15 a.m. and picked up my pen and logged the time as I answered the call, just as I had watched the drivers do.

'What time is surgery?' A hard-sounding woman's voice asked.

'Two until five in the afternoons,' I replied.

The phone went down without a word of thanks and I started to wonder what sort of person rang after midnight for surgery hours. I didn't have a lot of time to come up with any conclusions, as the phone went again. A nasal male voice this time, sounding like a character from Monty Python. 'I wonder if you can help me.' (Talking about the call a few nights later to Roy and Andy, they laughed out loud – apparently it was a sentence that often led to 'grief' as they put it.)

'If I can,' I replied, 'What seems to be the problem?'

The question was ignored. 'Got a pen? Take this number down.' The whining voice proceeded to give me an address in the depths of the East End of London.

'Hang on a minute,' I said. 'You haven't told me the problem yet.'

An edge appeared to the whine. ''E's limpin' on his front leg.'

'How long has he been limping?'

'About six weeks, but 'e's been getting worse. I want the vet out – now.'

'We don't do house visits. You'll have to bring him down to us. The surgery times are two till five in the afternoon.'

'Are you telling me you're refusing to treat my suffering dog?'

'We only see emergencies at this time of night,' I went on, starting to get an inkling of how Bill's heart attack may have been caused.

247

'This is an emergency.'

'No it isn't. You've already told me he's been limping for six weeks. Bring him in tomorrow,' and I went to put the phone down.

''Ere. Don't think you can hang up on me and get away with it you little toerag.' There followed an eruption of foul language and threats to report me to everyone the caller could think of, followed by demands to know my name and advice that I was going to be 'done over'.

I was shaking when I finally put the phone down. I couldn't believe it. First the woman with the puppy in the waiting room, now this. I was relieved to hear the sound of Andy driving his van into the car park.

If I thought he would be outraged, I was mistaken. He just shrugged his shoulders. 'You get used to it,' he said. 'Nine times out of ten when you get to meet these people they're small, insignificant and meek and mild to your face.' And he pointed out that we had more to worry about that evening than belligerent callers. He and Bill had worked together for a good few years.

The phone went again. This time Andy took it. It was the whiner again.

Andy listened intently and came out with what I had come to recognize as his stock phrase with difficult customers. 'Listen, friend, my colleague had already told you to come later on today. Please note that I said today. It is gone two in the morning. A few more hours will make no difference.'

The phone went down again, but not before Andy had got all the details of the caller. If he turned up tomorrow I would make sure it was me he saw.

For the first time since we had met, Andy and I didn't talk, but just sat quietly absorbed with our own thoughts and memories of Bill. 'I suppose he could die,' I said.

'Are you afraid of death?' Andy asked me.

'Aren't you?'

'No, I don't think so. That's where Buddhism helps. Have you heard of *nang pa*?'

I shook my head.

'It means "insider", someone who seeks the truth not outside but within the nature of his or her mind. All the teachings and training in Buddhism are aimed are at that one single point to look into the nature of mind and so free us from the fear of death and help us realize the truth of life.'

I couldn't sleep so I drove round to the hospital to see if I could find out any information. It was bedlam. There were four or five men with fight wounds, eyes clogged up with blood, hair matted, all drunk. And a couple of road traffic victims, who if their sobbing companions were anything to go by were probably drunk too. The casualty sister, a beacon of calm, told me that Bill was comfortable, that he'd had a coronary and was being well looked after in intensive care.

I drove back to the Harmsworth where it was all quiet, in total contrast to the nightmare scenario I had just left. It was 3.30 and I suddenly felt an overwhelming tiredness. I thought back to the previous night when I had been downing far too much alcohol myself, in an unknown flat in Mayfair.

'Call me if you need anyone on the phones again,' I said to Andy on my way back upstairs. 'But I'm bushed.' He gave me a wave. He was reading a book.

Up one flight of stairs, through the front door up the corridor and into bed, it took two minutes to get undressed and another two to be fast asleep.

I woke at ten to nine but still made it by nine after a quick shower. Andy was on the phone as I went past the night staff room.

'Any news from the hospital?' I asked.

'Looks like he'll pull through. I've just spoken to Phyllis. She's been with him since about six. One of her sons drove her up. They're a tight-knit family.'

I nodded and made my way downstairs and thought about what Andy had said last night. Was I afraid of death? Well I didn't want to die and more particularly at the moment I didn't want Bill to die. I said a prayer and walked bleary-eyed into the operating theatre.

I made it just before the boss himself walked in. 'I thought I sent you to back to bed for a decent sleep yesterday,' he said, staring at me. 'Yet you look as though you've come through a bush backwards. What happened?'

I filled him in on the night's dramas.

'Right. Back to bed with you. I'll do your stint in theatre this morning – all the office work is up to date. You'll need your energy for the afternoon – especially if Mr Nasty from last night turns up.'

Once again, who was I to argue with the boss? So I set the alarm for 12.30 and went back to bed. He was right – I was still very tired and sleep came almost immediately.

Mr Nasty, as Tony had named the whiner, turned out to be a wiry, wrinkled old man who produced a bus pass as proof of his age. I couldn't believe that the blood-curdling threats and oaths had come from this subservient OAP who was apologizing for ''avin a go' at one of the staff last night. I hadn't the energy to tell him it was me.

' I'd 'ad a skinful, know what I mean?' he said by way of mitigation. His dog, a Staffordshire bull terrier, submitted to an examination without any fuss. A nail had grown too long and was pressing on the pad. Fortunately it hadn't grown into the pad, as so often happens, but it would be uncomfortable to walk on – hence the limp.

'How long has he been limping?' I asked as I clipped the nail back, immediately relieving the pressure.

'Only a few days.'

'That wasn't what you said last night.'

He looked at me strangely. I took no notice.

A minute later the dog was walking around, sniffing the furniture.

''Ere. You've done a terrific job. Bloody brilliant. 'E's cured!'

Rizla, as he was called, danced on all four paws to prove the point. I looked at the bundle of cards belonging to animals waiting to see me. About twenty to go I reckoned. 'Come back if you're worried,' I said, and gave the old boy a card with our consulting times on it. 'And don't threaten me with a doing over next time.'

He opened his mouth in surprise, the truth suddenly dawning, but the next patient was already being ushered in and I gave him no chance to continue the discussion.

By 5.30 we were done and I went straight round to the hospital to see how Bill was doing. He was out of intensive care but the ward sister said she thought it would be better if I didn't go in to see him. It was a bit crowded, she said with his wife and all four sons. But it looked as if he would pull through.

On my way back to the flat I dropped in on Andy and Roy to report back. It was still early and the phones were quiet.

'Just as there's a strong link between stress and illness,' Andy said, 'there's a similar link between a strong belief structure and recovery.'

'But you could hardly call Bill a religious kind of bloke,' Roy chipped in.

'Belief is not necessarily to do with religion,' Andy explained. 'A strong sense of purpose is enough. The Viennese psychiatrist Victor Franko, who was himself a survivor of Auschwitz, discovered that the ones who survived the camps tended to be the ones with some deep faith or some overriding purpose in their lives.'

'So family could do it?' said Roy.

'Exactly. Something or someone we deeply love, that gives us some sense of higher purpose or direction.'

But family or no family, it was a good few months before Bill was back in harness again. Sadly he did not live to have a long retirement.

Chapter Sixteen

The week Tony was in Switzerland I scanned the weather maps at the back of the paper. It still rankled that he had gone and not me. Snow conditions had never interested me before; now I read them as avidly as the cricket scores.

Although during the six months I had been at the Harmsworth I had become used to the general run of cat and dog accidents and diseases, my experience of other animals was still limited to what chanced to come through the door. One evening when I was on evening duty I was faced for the first time with a tortoise, who had been rushed to the Harmsworth as an emergency.

Albert had been in the Sear family for years – handed down from generation to generation. He was thought to be at least sixty years old, although he was only small. Every year, regular as clockwork, he would stagger out of hibernation and meander about the garden, picking at bits and pieces of leaves and accepting cucumber and anything else the family offered him. He was always slow to eat and the family had got used to him gradually warming up and pottering about. This spring he was in for a shock, however.

Since Albert had gone to sleep in the autumn, the Sears had got another pet – an old English sheepdog no less, and very exuberant too. Dusty had been rescued from a family that had lost interest in her – they had probably bought her just because she looked cuddly when she was a puppy, but as soon as she started becoming a handful she'd been left locked up in a flat all day. Now just over a year old, she had never been trained and rushed around like a mad thing most of the time. The garden, Angela Sear told me, was beginning to look dishevelled, with most of her plants dug up and the lawn getting very patchy with the dog peeing everywhere.

The two Sear children spent a lot of time throwing a ball which Dusty would chase after, crashing through various plants to retrieve it. Nor was the family car faring too well. Dusty's speciality was eating the back seats in a frenzy of anticipation every time she was taken for a ride – she knew it heralded a nice long walk and she signalled her joy with a flurry of chewy activity.

Dusty did not pay much attention to Albert. She sniffed and pawed him when she first met him not long after he first came out of hibernation but soon lost interest in him once he retreated into his shell, which he very quickly learned to do.

This particular evening the children were playing with her in the garden. Dusty had found a smelly old slipper and was carrying it around in her mouth. One of the children had snatched it from her and threw it. This was a fine game and Dusty took after it like a greyhound. It landed on top of poor old Albert, who must have wondered what hit him because Dusty grabbed both slipper and Albert, throwing both about, before racing up to the children and proudly depositing Albert at their feet. To their horror Dusty's teeth had made a gaping hole in his shell. He was put in a box and rushed down to the hospital in the middle of my evening emergency clinic.

It was just starting to get dark when they arrived *en famille*, in a great state of panic. Fortunately Trevor hadn't set off for home – he was tinkering with his car in the car park, adjusting the carburettor. Although I knew nothing about tortoises, I knew that Trevor did, having inherited one from Susannah's family. We had been talking about it only a day or so before, as he had just become one of the first members of the British Chelonian Society. If I'd been asked a week earlier what a chelonian was, I wouldn't have had a clue.

We were soon gently bathing Albert's wounds with povidone iodine, the solution we used to scrub up with before doing operations. The tortoise seemed remarkably alert. 'Good thing he doesn't seem too shocked,' Trevor remarked. 'I wouldn't fancy trying to set up a drip on him.'

The plan was quite straightforward. We would keep him in for three or four days bathing his wounds daily and dosing him with antibiotics to prevent any infection, and then he would need the shell fixed. 'How?' was my immediate question – I had given up any pretence of knowledge I did not have.

But Trevor said he wasn't sure either. He'd consult with the experts, other members of the Chelonian Society. Anyway the wounds needed time to heal first.

Tony returned from Switzerland as pale as when he had left a week before. Trevor was right, he hadn't set a foot outside the conference hotel. The lectures had been 'fantastic', he said, and he couldn't wait to buy the system for the Harmsworth. I had never seen him so fired up. A flurry of memos were sent to headquarters and during the breaks he could be seen on the phone in his office trying to arrange the finance. Things began to happen quickly. First to arrive was a huge oxygen cylinder, then the equipment itself, which came in two stainless steel boxes which could have doubled as canteen food containers.

Watching him going through them was like watching a

kid at Christmas. 'The object of the exercise,' he said as he went through the procedure with us a couple of days later, 'is to push the two broken bones together, under pressure compression, so that they heal rapidly and the leg gets back to normal straight away, thus avoiding the stiffening-up usually associated with fracture disease.'

The good news was that we would all need to understand the new procedure, and Tony had promised to book Trevor and me onto the first available course. In the meantime we had other things to mend, and about a week later I discovered Trevor in the prep room bent over Albert the tortoise. 'So, you've come up with an answer then.'

'I have, Maestro. Epoxy resin. Araldite to you.'

DIY was a great forte of Trevor's, having spent most of the last six months completely redecorating a dilapidated house he had just bought and in the process doubling its value. Living above the hospital it never occurred to me to buy property and as a result I missed out on the first great property-value explosions that occurred in the seventies.

The Sears picked up Albert the next day. They had already fenced off a portion of garden exclusively for him. As with most of the accidents that I was to see, the lesson was learned and steps taken to prevent it happening again.

For the next few months, every fracture case was pounced upon by Tony almost as it hobbled, limped or hopped through the door. We got used to the high-pitched whine of the air drill as it made holes in the bone for the screws that would hold the plates together.

I was the first to spot the next course – or so I thought when I knocked on Tony's office door one morning in May with the *Veterinary Record* in my hand. But he had been there before me.

'Quite so. I've already booked you and Trevor in,' he

said. 'They've managed to compress the course into three days because there won't be any possibility of skiing.'

Quite right, I thought. It doesn't snow very often in June in Potters Bar.

For both Trevor and me, there was a sense of *déjà vu* as we enrolled at reception, because this was our alma mater, the Royal Veterinary College. The lecturers were the same as on the Davos course: a world-famous human orthopaedic surgeon from New York, an American veterinary surgeon, a Canadian and four Swiss orthopaedic surgeons who apparently flew themselves into Hatfield airport in their own private planes.

It had been four years since I had last attended anything this concentrated, but soon I was in the swing of things. There was a great contrast between the charismatic, live-wire wise-cracking Americans and the reflective Swiss, with their sing-song German accents. Because a lot of 'shop' was talked well into the night, we were never in bed before two, but by 8.30 in the morning were back at our desks, raring to go. I finally learned that most basic of lessons – that the more you put in, the more you get out. Better late than never.

Then it was back to work on Monday with a spring in my step and a sneaky glance down the operations list to bag the fractures before Trevor got in. But it was a classic case of Murphy's law: for what was probably the first time since the hospital opened there were no fractures awaiting repair.

I didn't have long to wait for my first case, however. As Tony had covered for us all weekend, Trevor elected to do Monday night, so I got Tuesday. It was just before midnight that Roy got the call: a Labrador out for its last walk with its owner before going to bed had been hit on a zebra crossing by a speeding car – which proceeded to drive off at an even greater speed. The dog was hit in the front leg. Both he and his shocked owner – a teenager who was looking after him while his parents were on holiday – were brought into the Harmsworth by a police patrol car called to the scene by a witness.

Jasper was one of those phlegmatic dogs typical of his breed. Although he must have been in considerable pain he submitted to my examination with no more than a reproachful look. The bone was obviously broken, but he didn't seem to be suffering from shock, which could not be said for the boy, who was so shaken up the policemen were debating whether to take him to Casualty. Although he was shaking, however, he made clear that he was going nowhere until he was sure that the dog was all right. So Roy made him a cup of tea and wrapped him in a blanket while Andy and I set about doing the preliminary work on the black Labrador.

It was a fairly straightforward case; Jasper's right front leg was broken in two about halfway up. He flinched slightly when I touched it and nuzzled my hand away, then sat quietly on the table while I took an X-ray, which showed a clean break right through the radius and ulna.

It was not long since a new type of gutter splint had made its way onto the market. It was plastic and moulded to fit a dog's leg and, lined with foam rubber, was excellent. Moreover, if you were gentle, it could be fitted with the dog still awake. While Andy held Jasper's head, I put the splint around the broken leg and bandaged it up. I could sense the dog's relief immediately and when Roy brought in his young owner Jasper was completely relaxed and wagging his tail. 'As you can see, he's fine, at least for the time being,' I explained to the boy. 'But he'll need an operation in the morning.'

I was up very early for a change, to bag the operation before anyone else could, and I asked Mary if she was free to be the nurse assisting. It all went like clockwork. I cut down to the broken bones, got them back into position and put the plate on. To the uninitiated it must have looked like basic carpentry – albeit in sterile conditions – and consisted of drilling nine holes into the bone which would to take the screws that would keep the plate in place.

An hour and a half later Mary was developing the post-operative X-ray. This is always the acid test, but she came out beaming. 'Not bad for a beginner,' she said, handing over the negative. And there it was, plate and screws sitting snugly against the bone, and you couldn't even see where the break had been. And there was better to come: the next day Jasper was already putting weight on the leg and the day after, Tony sent him home. I would have liked him to stay in for a further week so that I could keep an eye on him and follow the progress of my first bone-fixing patient, but, as Tony was quick to remind me, the best place for any animal to recover is at home.

Two weeks later Jasper came back for a check-up, and I felt a certain amount of pride when I saw him walking normally. The main danger now was that the owner would forget to rest him for another month, but fortunately young Jonathan showed sense beyond his years and the dog went on to make a complete recovery.

We found out later that a quick-witted motorist had seen the accident and noted the registration number of the speeding car. The driver was later arrested and prosecuted for failing to stop after an accident. A perfect ending.

It seemed with some people though, that the lesson was never learned. Weasel was a smallish crossbred dog with a fracture of his radius and ulna. He had been run over two days before and after being stabilized for shock had been X-rayed. I had grabbed the case before Trevor had got in – one of the advantages of living over the shop. The operation had gone without a hitch and I left the writing up of the notes to Mary. I had been working quite a lot with her recently, as Tony was getting bogged down with more and more paperwork and Trevor and I were only too keen to get stuck in.

'Look at this!' I heard her exclaim as she was writing on the clinical card. 'The poor dog's only ten months old and this is the third accident he's had. Looks like you know his owner.' There written on the card was a warning to the owner, Mrs Norton, in my handwriting, to keep the dog under control and the reply to 'keep my nose right out of it'.

I hadn't recognized Weasel as the puppy I had seen a few months before. Already he'd had three accidents. The first just needed a few stitches, but the second resulted in a broken leg which because he was so young – only five months, only needed a plaster of Paris. This latest was the most serious, needing internal fixation.

'I'll talk to her when she comes in to pick him up,' said Mary, and I knew that this would be more likely to produce results than a talking to from me. Mrs Norton simply had no respect for young men, whereas Mary carried an aura about her which meant that few dared to cross her.

A few days later Mary mentioned to me that she didn't think she had got anywhere with Weasel's owner. 'A tough nut if ever I saw one. She spent most of the time looking out of the window,' she said. 'Obviously wasn't listening. She didn't even bother to bring a lead to walk him to the car.'

It was a time when lots of people seemed to be careless when out with their dogs. Most days there were three of four fracture cases in – so many that Trevor and I didn't even try to bag them any more, there were plenty to go round. Every day the operating theatre resounded to the sound of the electric drill as one of us spent hours on end putting broken bones together. Thirty years later I get the impression that people are more careful. For the most part, though, most animals only had one accident and then their owners learned their lesson. Mrs Norton was an exception.

I arrived one morning to find Trevor bent over a young dog that had been involved in an RTA earlier in the day. He had been called out and had spent the last hour and a half battling to save the dog's life. It was a battle that was lost just as I arrived. 'Both front legs have been broken and he's got a ruptured spleen. His right eye would have had to come out and the jaw's broken. Poor little mite. No ID. I wonder who he belongs to. It's obviously happened before,' he added.

'Look,' I said, pointing to the X-ray clipped up behind him. 'There's a plate and screws in the radius and ulna.' These are the bones between the elbow and the carpus, what in humans we call the forearm.

Just then Mary came in with Tony, ready to do the ward rounds. 'I'm surprised at you, Mr Grant. You should recognize that dog. It's your handiwork,' she said, looking at the plate on the X-Ray, then towards the dead animal on the operating table. 'It's Weasel isn't it?' Like many of the nurses who spent hours nursing a dog that I had spent only one hour operating on, she had a photographic memory for patients months after they had gone home.

She came back a few moments later with Mrs Norton's card. It was Weasel right enough. He had been knocked down right outside her house, yet we hadn't heard from her.

'I'll give her a call and say we think her dog's in here,' said Trevor. He came back a few minutes later, looking grim-faced. 'She's on her way.'

As Weasel's owner was brought through to the prep room no attempt was made to clean up the blood on his face and elsewhere, or to remove the drips that had been set up. She clasped her hand to her mouth in horror when she saw her dog.

'I did my best,' said Trevor. 'Pity you didn't do yours. Make sure you don't get another dog.' And with that she was led out. No cockiness this time, just averted eyes. I felt no sorrow for her, only for latch-key Weasel. Four accidents in less than a year – the last one fatal.

Life at the Harmsworth went on. The cases we saw were very similar to those that I had encountered in Canterbury, but it was the people I came across who stuck in my mind. One in particular, Molly Parsons, managed to confound every expectation.

It was a day in early July, hot and sweaty as only London can be. Londoners are great ones for enjoying the sun at every opportunity and the Harmsworth's clients were no different. I arrived to find the car park full of men and women stripped off for the beach, waiting for surgery to begin. The waiting room in contrast was practically empty, except for a slightly plump Marilyn Monroe lookalike with startling long blonde hair and a low-cut sundress. As Trevor and I ploughed through the afternoon's appointments, we grinned at each from time to time at each other wondering who would get 'Marilyn'.

'What's that smell?' I said to him as an aside as we passed in the corridor with respective owners.

'What, my after shave? Or do you mean essence of ferret?'

'Ferret?' A wave of mild panic engulfed me. 'I don't know anything about ferrets.'

Still Practising

'Don't worry about it,' he said. 'They're quite simple to treat, just nip next door if you get her,' he added nodding in the direction of 'Marilyn', 'and I'll fill you in.'

When I put my head into the waiting room and called out Molly Parsons, the blonde jumped up with a smile on her face. She coughed loudly. 'It's not only Johnny 'as got the flu. I reckon you'll 'ave to see to me an' all,' and she followed me into the consulting room.

I looked at the clinical record. Johnny was the ferret. However I could see no sign of anything that might contain an animal: no pram, no push-chair, not even a vacuum cleaner.

'Where is he?' I asked.

In answer she began to wriggle and move her hips like a hoola dancer and moved her arms behind her back. A lump appeared in her midriff and she began to bounce up and down, pushing it up. Then her substantial bosom did a sudden heave and a blonde furry head popped out, as did my eyes. The ferret gave me a pink-eyed stare, then dived back into the sanctuary of Marilyn's midriff. She immediately started the bouncing routine again, which had the effect of making her ample bosom wobble like a gigantic jelly. The head appeared again.

'I can't manage this on me own,' said Molly. 'Grab 'is 'ead.'

I was dimly aware of a couple of nurses and Trevor looking through the hatch between the surgeries, enjoying the spectacle. I made a grab at Johnny but he was too quick and to my utter embarrassment I was suddenly aware of my hand being halfway down Molly's cleavage.

Ferrets are one of the more unlikely pets I have encountered in my time. An albino form of polecat, they have been bred in captivity for at least 1500 years and

263

appeared in Britain around the time of the Norman conquest. Originally used for hunting rabbits, now they're as likely to be owned by young women who like to have a furry cuddly thing to carry around with them. However, they have one major drawback, their remarkable smell, which though it cannot be described, also cannot be forgotten, and it beats me how the owners put up with it.

'Let's try again, shall we Doc,' said Molly with an even bigger smile than before, but I felt discretion was the better part of valour and got Karen, who I knew was in the prep room, to come and give me a hand. She managed to snare Johnny's head and I got hold of him behind his neck and hauled him out.

'So,' I said, feeling distinctly hot and bothered. 'What seems to be the problem?'

''E's got the flu, same as me. I read it in one of me books,' and as if to illustrate the point Molly launched into a paroxysm of coughing which was only brought to a halt by a similar outbreak from Johnny. 'What did I tell you,' she simpered. ''E's got it from me.'

Having never handled a ferret before I was extremely apprehensive. Johnny proved surprisingly amenable, however. He was very tame and let me take his temperature. He had runny eyes and a runny nose, and generally looked a bit seedy. Perhaps Molly's homespun diagnosis was right. 'He does look a bit fluey, I have to say. But just give me a minute, I'll have a word with my colleague.'

'Could be,' Trevor was quick to confirm. 'Ferrets can get our flu, and we can get it from them. Don't ask me to examine him – or her,' he added with a grin. 'You seem to have picked up the bedside manner pretty quickly. You must remember to put "dab hand in ferret retrieval" on your CV.'

'What do you treat it with?' I asked, ignoring his attempt at humour.

'Same as you would treat yourself. Good nursing. Antibiotics are no use – it's a virus.'

I went back into the consulting room but Johnny had disappeared back into his sanctuary.

'He just needs good nursing. He should be as right as rain in a week – and so should you. But you have to watch out for pneumonia, both of you.'

'What about examining me?' said Molly.

'You'll need to go to your doctor for that,' I said firmly. She had been making as if to undo the buttons on her blouse.

'Only joking. I'm going to put myself to bed with a warm hot water bottle.'

'Just what I was going to suggest,' I replied.

'You don't do home visits do you?'

'Afraid not – too busy here. Make sure you keep him warm.'

'No problem – he always sleeps with me,' she winked.

At which Johnny popped his head up and sneezed a fine spray of virus particles in my face.

Chapter Seventeen

As soon as I joined the RSPCA I became aware of Club Row, a street market that operated every Sunday in London's East End, where animals were bought and sold under conditions that didn't bear thinking about. Although the dealers had to be licensed by the local authority, the standards were very low and many a time the RSPCA were called in to pick up puppies and kittens abandoned because they hadn't been sold by the end of the day.

Over the years many an inspector had tried to close Club Row down. None had succeeded, although individual traders did lose their licences from time. But Jim Halliwell was cast from a different mould. By the time I met him, he was in his late thirties. Before joining the RSPCA he'd been a commando and seen action in the Korean War. In many ways, his experiences as a commando made him the best sort of person to take on the challenges of his East End patch: he was utterly fearless and relished a fight.

The nature of his 'patch' meant that he came across more than his fair share of cruelty cases, and he pursued them like a detective might pursue a murderer, with a tenacity that made him work hours on end. And he got results, clocking up more than double the average number of prosecutions every year.

Jim was every inch a soldier, built like a tank and as broad as he was tall. He had a neck like an ox, so thick it merged into his shoulders. Without the day-to-day intensive physical training of the Army, he had begun to put on weight, but he still managed to exude an air of aggression which protected him from up-front abuse. He was obsessed by Club Row. Every Sunday he was down there in his uniform on the look out for any sick animals that shouldn't be on sale, and he would hang around and warn people if they were contemplating buying anything to be careful, especially if so-called pedigrees were being offered.

But the nature of these markets, selling very young animals, is that they have a built-in vulnerability factor and once punters, as the traders called the customers, had set their hearts on little Rover or Tiddles, then all Jim could do was to warn them that it wasn't a good idea to buy anything without a pedigree and not to part with cash. 'Get the animal checked by a vet before you pay anything,' was his motto and he had the names of local vets who ran Sunday surgeries.

Naturally neither his intervention nor his presence was popular with the numerous stall-holders. On one occasion he told me how he had arrived in the early morning and had had a tin of dog food hurled at him. His response was to pick it up, smile at the group of dealers who were responsible and tell them he knew an old-age pensioner with a dog who would be grateful for their generosity.

A tin of dog food is one thing, death threats are another, and Jim had his share of those, but he would repeat them as someone else might tell a joke. Like the time his wife answered the door to discover a hearse and two undertakers saying they'd come for 'the late Jim Halliwell'. 'I told them they were a bit premature. That I was still very much alive and to pass the message on to whoever was paying them.'

I found some of his stories incredible until I had first-hand experience myself.

Trevor and I were ploughing through the usual Monday afternoon mass of clinic cases. By this time I was up to speed and could match him for efficiency and clinical accuracy. I had quickly learned that most of the cases were routine and would get better quite quickly with simple treatments. Anything complicated would be admitted for further investigation. It was a system which by and large worked; the only times when things went seriously wrong were when people brought in lots of animals at one time – one of Bridey Donovan's favourite tricks – and the occasional irate customer who might need a bit of time to be calmed down.

This particular Monday afternoon was going well and the waiting room was beginning to empty out. Just as well – it was a hot sticky summer's afternoon with the clients sitting in the equivalent of a sauna. A row started up between a young man and a middle-aged woman who was berating him for keeping a puppy in a sweaty, smelly old duffel bag in such hot weather. As voices were raised, I went out to see what was happening. As they were the last two of the day, I took the man and Trevor took the woman.

Joe had bought the puppy the day before, he told me, 'off a man in a pub' and wanted to get it vaccinated. It was for his girlfriend, a surprise. She had always wanted a corgi, 'because of the Queen'. He had gone to Club Row because he'd heard of it, but there were no corgis anywhere. Eventually one dealer said he thought he knew where he could get one and to wait in the pub and he'd see what he could do.

Joe was just about to give up when the dealer returned with the duffel bag. The pup was young, a bit too young really, the dealer explained, but this little rascal was eating like an eight-week old. 'And you've got a bargain,' the stall-holder had said, 'his father was a Crufts champion.' The young man had been persuaded to hand over £50 – 'half-price'. This was a lot of money, several weeks' wages for someone like Joe.

When Joe asked to hold him, the man had acted conspiratorially, said it was against the rules to sell except in the street as a licensed trader, but gave him a quick look at the sleek brindle coat. As for the corgi's papers, no problem, the man had said. He could send them on to Joe when the rest of the litter were registered by the Kennel Club in a couple of weeks. He could keep the duffel bag, he said. 'Be a shame to wake the little blighter up.' He also gave him a tin of dog food that would do till he got some in the morning. His parting shot was apparently, 'I'll be seeing you in Crufts in a year or two.'

Joe had put his hand in the bag and felt the warm creature stir as he stroked it. He could hardly believe his luck. A future Crufts champion for only £50! Naturally he didn't want to take risks with his investment, hence the need for vaccinations.

'So what have you been feeding him on?' I asked.

'Pedigree Chum.'

I told him that wouldn't do and that he'd need to get special puppy food. I also told him that at six weeks he was too young for vaccination. But we could worm him. Dealers are notoriously unwilling to spend money on anything they don't have to. It was only then that I asked to see the puppy.

It had a bushy tail and a very long snout. I stared at it, hardly able to believe my eyes. This was one eventuality that my training had singularly failed to prepare me for. But there was no way to soften the blow. 'I'm sorry to tell you,' I said. 'But this isn't a corgi. It's a fox cub.'

I will never forget the look that came into Joe's eyes:

David Grant

open-eyed bewilderment followed by narrow-eyed anger. Anger not directed at the dealer, I soon discovered, but at me.

I repeated what I had said. 'It's a fox cub.'

'Nah, nah,' Joe said pushing the cub back into the duffel bag. 'It's a corgi. You don't know what you're talking about. Think I'm stupid or somefing?'

I just shook my head.

'I want a second opinion!'

I caught sight of Karen's face at the dispensing hatch – she had been disturbed by the sound of Joe's rising voice. 'Karen, will you ask Trevor to come in for a minute?'

Trevor had always had quite an interest in wildlife, having operated on birds to fix broken wings, and was generally reckoned to be the in-house expert. He came in with a puzzled look on his face, wondering what all the commotion was about. Initially on hearing the shouting, he had wondered if it was just another drunk. At the time the pubs used to shut at three in the afternoon and often an animal's owner would come straight from the pub, well under the influence of drink, into the waiting room. But Joe was not drunk – just angry.

'What do you think of this little chap?' I asked.

Trevor carefully examined the animal. He had plenty of experience in dealing with potentially tricky situations and wasn't going to rush anything. Not that he had any idea of the background at this stage at all. 'Lovely little fellow.' he said, 'But very young.' Then he turned to Joe. 'Where did you find him? He needs to go back to his mother. Back to the wild. Fox cubs don't do well in captivity.'

'You give 'im here. He's a corgi!' stormed Joe, snatching the dozing creature back from Trevor. 'I paid good money for him. I'm going to get another opinion –

from a proper vet.' With that he put the cub back in the duffel bag and without saying a further word left the building.

Later, over a pint, Trevor told me another story, equally unlikely. 'This bloke buys a golden Labrador puppy in a pub. Takes it right away to his local vet. So far so good. Then, after taking the history and discussing diet and all that, the vet gets the pup out of the basket and it turns out to be a very large overweight hamster!' I nearly choked on my beer.

At this point we were joined by Jim Halliwell who had just come off duty and had heard about the commotion in the waiting room. Naturally, this being his special area, he had come to find us for the low down. He was interested in following the story up – particularly if it could be linked to any particular trader. Part of his campaign was directed at the out-and-out villains to get their licences to trade revoked. He laughed at the hamster story. 'Haven't heard that one before,' he said. 'Though I'm not saying it's not true. Very little surprises me now. It's a lethal combination: villains so fly they would sell their grandmother if they thought they could make a killing and a gullible public who'd buy Bambi if they could fit her into a paper bag.'

He told us another Labrador story, one which had happened to him so he could vouch for its authenticity. One Sunday he had been down in Club Row and had noticed a couple with a young child looking at Labrador puppies. He had first talked to the woman, with his usual line of not parting with cash before seeing the pedigree papers. She had taken no notice, of course. But he had overheard the conversation that followed. The woman didn't want a bitch because of the nuisance, as she saw it, of coming into season. Then she saw one that she liked the look of. Was it definitely a dog, she had asked the trader? Yes. And he pointed underneath to the dog's penis.

'Now by chance I had seen those labs a while earlier and I knew they were all bitches. What the trader had done was push her tail between her legs and alongside the belly. That's what he was pointing at.'

'So what happened then?'

'I stepped in and the dealer had to admit it. But you'll never believe what. They bought it anyway. Fallen in love with it. Suddenly it didn't matter what sex it was.

'Got your roster for the weekend lads?' he continued. 'Know who's on duty this Sunday?'

'I am,' I said.

'Right, well, this is something that might interest you, David, broaden your practical experience. I'm planning a raid in Club Row and, all being well, I shall need a hand.'

'Count me in.'

I promptly forgot about the raid, dismissing it as Jim's bluster. I had misjudged him. At 10.30 the following Sunday I was just finishing ward rounds when one of the nurses on duty with me came through to the back of the hospital to tell me that Inspector Halliwell had arrived with a van full of cats and dogs – five kittens and five puppies to be precise. All were by his own reckoning suffering from infectious diseases, so one by one they were trundled through to the prep room for a physical examination.

Every detail had to be meticulously recorded because this was the only written evidence that would be admissible in court. A court case would certainly be following and, knowing my inexperience, Jim took great pains to ensure that everything was done by the book.

The five kittens were all straightforward enough. All had

runny noses, temperatures and runny eyes. Every now and then one would sneeze – nothing like our sneezes, just a short, sharp sound like someone saying a 't' sound. They had flu and were not fit for sale. Were they suffering enough to satisfy a court of law? Apparently they were on sale in the open air – the stall-holder would later maintain that this was for better ventilation because he thought they had a 'slight' cold. ('Nuffin wrong wiv a bit of fresh air yer honour.') It was enough for me to feel comfortable about writing out a certificate stating that the kittens had suffered unnecessarily.

The puppies, mongrels – Labrador/spaniel cross I should judge – were more complex, however. They had all the signs of distemper, although if I were right, it would be the first time I had come across this horrible disease. They too were all coughing with runny noses.

Although it starts innocently enough, with the symptoms of a cold, distemper is one of the most distressing diseases a dog can get. It's a virus infection, a bit like polio in humans. Not only is there the danger of the dog developing pneumonia, but after about three or four weeks it affects the nervous system; some dogs get nervous twitching of the muscles and others develop a form of epilepsy. There is no cure, because the damage to the nerves is permanent. To prevent this horrible disease, puppies should be vaccinated at about eight weeks. If I was right, these puppies, like so many on sale at Club Row, had clearly not been vaccinated.

Distemper is extremely contagious and for obvious reasons I was unhappy about keeping them in the hospital. So after cleaning them up they were transported across to a private vet based outside London. John Robinson had done innumerable cruelty cases for the RSPCA and was generally reckoned to be a dog expert.

David Grant

'We've got him,' said Jim as he prepared to set off with
the puppies to drive to Robinson's house in the country.
'Him' was one Reg Garner, a man whom Jim described as
'the Moriarty of the animal world'. Jim was like a man
possessed. Red in the face and with his hat pulled even
further down his head than usual, he headed off, leaving us
to take care of the kittens and saying he'd be back in the
morning to collect my statement.

I got the nurse on duty to clean the kittens' noses and
give them all antibiotics while I hurried upstairs where
Gloria 2 had a Colombian bean stew waiting for me. I had
taken to these after visiting Henry and Berta's house. It
seemed they featured in a lot of Colombian recipes. It was
the first time that my kitchen had seen any cooking beyond
a fry-up and the odd tin-opening. The smells were
tantalizing and when I got in she was busy laying the table:
flowers, napkins, a salad bowl – even warm plates and a
saucepan full with *frijoles* – Spanish for kidney beans that
had been soaked for twenty four hours prior to cooking.

Gloria poured out a cold Spanish beer – San Miguel. It
was the nearest she could get to the real thing. Apparently
Colombians weren't into wine with meals as much as lager.
The national drink was aguardiente which seemed to be
almost identical to Greek ouzo. I couldn't have aguardiente
today because I was on duty and I had already found out it
was pretty lethal stuff.

To Gloria it seemed a bit quaint that such a hullabaloo
should be caused by a market selling kittens and puppies
that weren't healthy. 'I tell you, David, in Colombia
children are treated worse than you British treat your
animals. I know it is your job, but isn't all this fuss just a bit
ridiculous?'

After lunch I decided to take her down to see the kittens

274

in the isolation unit. And as soon as she saw them, of course, her attitude changed. They had been cleaned up, fleas had been combed from them and soothing ointment had been put in their eyes. It was as much as I could do to stop her taking them home there and then. They would have to stay at the Harmsworth for a week or so until somewhere else could be found for them. Meanwhile, they would get intensive treatment and their whereabouts kept secret. Jim Halliwell had no doubts that if the stall-owner knew they were at the hospital he would try to get them back by fair means or foul. They were evidence. Officially no one knew they were under our care. They were just called C/C Inspector Halliwell – C/C meaning cruelty case.

The next day he was back and with the help of the hospital secretary a Statement of Suffering was typed up. Every single detail of each kitten was recorded and finally the all-important statement that the kittens had suffered unnecessarily in my professional opinion. John Robinson had come to exactly the same conclusion about the puppies, and agreed with my diagnosis that they had distemper. Whereas our kittens would certainly get better, the same could not be said for these little scraps. They, unfortunately, had a very poor outlook.

The whole process of instigating legal proceedings is fraught with problems, and Reg Garner proved to be an elusive character. But he was eventually found, interviewed and subsequently prosecuted. The prosecution itself proved a long and tortuous business. On the first occasion Reg failed to turn up at the magistrates' court. He was later arrested and bailed to appear. This time he did show up but pleaded not guilty.

As the veterinary surgeon who had examined the kittens, I was called as an expert witness. The trial was held in Thames Court. There is something about courts that makes even the most innocent person feel nervous. I hadn't been charged with anything but I was as terrified as if I were on trial myself. Although I had seen numerous television plays and films and thought I knew what it would be like, when it came to standing up in the witness box, I found I could hardly speak, even though in many respects it was very low key, with just three magistrates sitting in judgement, none of them wearing the paraphernalia associated with British justice. Even now, when the number of such cases that I have done runs into the hundreds, the sense of responsibility turns me to jelly.

For all his not-guilty plea, Reg elected to say very little, and in the face of my evidence and Jim's, he was found guilty and given a fine of £200 with costs – a massive amount for that time. 'It's a diabolical liberty,' he shouted, announced that he would appeal, and duly did.

The appeal case was a very grand affair – or so it seemed to me at the time. I was warned that it would take all day in front of a judge. Witnesses came from all over the place including John Robinson, who had travelled from his country house in Wiltshire because the case started on a Monday morning. Whether it was because he couldn't find any self-respecting barrister to take him on, or was just feeling bloody-minded, Reg had decided to represent himself. This time his approach was quiet different from the last occasion and he had gone to great lengths to look professional. He was surrounded by sheaves of paper and tattered-looking books. The essence of his defence was that he knew best after thirty years of experience in the business, and that the vets were wrong, especially the young one who didn't look old enough to be a vet in the first place.

He reserved his most severe cross examination for me.

Quickly, however, he tied himself up in knots. He failed to understand the evidence, insisting that the kittens only had a slight cold 'like what humans get', and that they didn't have any symptoms of flu. He obviously didn't know what he was talking about and was constantly interrupted by the prosecuting barrister when he got hold of the wrong end of the stick.

The case finally wound up and the judge, an elderly, sharp-witted man resplendent in gown and wig, asked the defendant if he had anything to add. Reg launched into a passionate speech about how honest he was, how he was providing a service to the public, how he truly loved animals, and how he really understood their needs and wouldn't do anything to harm a hair on their innocent little heads – every sentiment interspersed with liberal helpings of 'yer honour'.

'Thank you,' said the judge. 'Appeal dismissed.'

At this there were immediate howls of rage from the considerable numbers of Reg's family and other supporters who had assembled in the public gallery. Several were ejected by the police. The various parties then jumped up to state their costs. John Robinson's costs came to more than £200 since he had claimed an hourly rate since leaving home first thing in the morning. The original fine was doubled, the costs were trebled and Reg was banned from keeping cats and dogs for the rest of his life.

As we left the court Jim was beaming; his chest, which even on a bad day was impressive, looked as though it was about to pop its buttons. It was, in the inspector's parlance, 'a good result', and he was bursting with glee. However, it didn't take long to work out that, to use Andy's phrase, it was a Pyrrhic victory and the Garners and their ilk would be even more careful to keep out of Jim's way. Reg himself

David Grant

might have had a body blow, but the ban was confined to him alone; it wouldn't stop Reg's family trading in animals. But Reg Garner was a key figure and the case of *Regina v Garner* was the first blow in a long war of attrition which was to lead eventually to the shutting down of the market.

After a celebratory pint with Jim Halliwell I made my back to the Harmsworth. On my way up to the flat I dropped in on Andy and Roy to give them the good news. They were often at the front line of cruelty cases and a victory, however small, was a victory nonetheless. I was pleased to see that Magda was with them, but she seemed strangely subdued as I retold the story of Reg Garner's downfall. I soon found out why.

'Bit of bad news, I'm afraid, David,' she said. 'Flo died last night. Massive stroke, they say.' Magda's old people were her family and I sensed that she wasn't just passing on information; she was truly upset and needed someone to share it with, someone who knew Flo. 'The funeral's set for next Tuesday. It'll be a real East End do. I wondered if you fancied coming?'

Why not, I thought.

'Course, you do know that they'll take you for my fancy man,' she chortled.

Flo Fountain's funeral was unlike anything I have ever seen. The horses pulling the hearse were decked out with black plumes and their manes were plaited with gold and black tassels. If respect was what Flo wanted, it was only a shame that she didn't see how they pushed the boat out for her at the end: Bentleys and Rolls-Royces and everyone kitted out in clothes that would not have been out of place at an investiture at Buckingham Palace. I even thought I might catch sight of Reg Garner or his family, but Magda said no. In the hierarchy of the East End Flo was aristocracy. Reg, she said, was just a small-time crook.

Magda was obviously known; nods were exchanged with all manner of people. 'There's so-and-so,' she would whisper with a knowing look, assuming I knew who she was talking about. And 'the old bill' were also much in evidence, she reported. No one missed a gangland funeral, she said, though there would be a few quick getaways as soon as the coffin was in the ground.

It struck me, as I sat with Magda at the back of the church, that she needed me beside her that day, just as Flo needed her sparklers. She gave her all, every day, to her animals and her "old dears", and like so many people who give unstintingly, Magda herself was taken for granted.

Seeing Henry's car parked behind the hospital when I returned, I went in to have a chat. Tony had brought him in to cover my absence. I hadn't seen him for some time, and an East End gangster funeral is not something he would ever have experienced, I reckoned. I found him in the prep room with an old tortoise shell Trevor had found for him to practise mending.

'So,' he said, after I had told him about the dark glasses and blacked-out windows of the limousines, 'What happened with the two Glorias?'

'I did as you told me and told Gloria No. 1 about Gloria No. 2 over an intimate – and very expensive – dinner. It was the least I could do to make up for having let things drift.'

'And?'

'And nothing.'

'But you did tell her?'

'Of course, but I found she knew already.'

It turned out that one evening months before she had phoned up to speak to me and Roy had said that I was on the phone talking to 'the other Gloria', so she had put two and two together. Roy had known ever since the beginning.

'That little whippersnapper needs a lesson in diplomacy,' Henry sighed.

'Maybe. But, come on, it was my fault really, as you pointed out.'

'So how did you leave it?'

'Just like it was. I told her that I never spoke Spanish with Gloria 2 and she seemed to like that. She sees herself as my mentor, not my lover. And you must understand Henry, that it was never really like that between us anyway.'

'Not even a little bit?'

'Not even a little bit. Anyway, she is determined that I should build on what I have learnt with her and that I should go to Colombia. She says she'll look into finding me a job there.'

He nearly dropped the shell. 'You're not serious?'

'Of course not, although it would be a wonderful opportunity. It would really give me a chance to come to grips with the language. Don't look so surprised – I take it you do have animals in Colombia?'

'We do, but not many ferrets, I have to say.' That was one incident I knew I would never live down. 'Though plenty of tropical birds.' Or that one.

I left Henry with his tube of Araldite and walked up to the flat. When I had first thought of becoming a vet I had thought it would give me an opportunity of working with animals, but I had had no idea that it would be a doorway into other worlds. First Canterbury, then London, which had given me an insight into the underbelly of that cosy English way of life that I had taken for granted before coming to the Harmsworth. South America was yet another world. Enticing though the thought of Colombia might be I had no intention of leaving the Harmsworth just yet. I had been there barely a year and the more I learned, the more I discovered there was to learn. I had just heard from Nick that he had handed in his notice in Canterbury. Two years was what he had said, and two years was what he had done. Two years was the minimum he said for anything to be of any practical use, three to really consolidate. Now he had taken a job in Devon where he came from, to consolidate his small-animal experience before moving into the world of academic veterinary research.

Meanwhile life for me was better than I had ever imagined it could be. There was a real sense at the Harmsworth of doing what I had always wanted to do – save lives – and if I did decide to go to Colombia at some point in the future, my Spanish would have to be better than it was now. In Gloria 1 I had the most elegant teacher, the best companion I could ever hope to have. And in Gloria 2 I had the most intoxicating girlfriend a man could wish for. Why would I want to leave all that? One of Andy's philosophers would probably have had an answer. But I preferred Dibber's Kentish philosophy when I asked him why he didn't marry Muriel, the lady friend who accompanied him on his foreign trips: 'If it ain't broke, don't mend it.'